Sybil D. Smith, PhD, RN
Editor

Parish Nursing
A Handbook
for the New Millennium

Pre-publication
REVIEWS,
COMMENTARIES,
EVALUATIONS . . .

This book is an excellent tool for parish nurses who are in active practice, but also for those who are thinking about this specialty in nursing. It not only gives the how to's but also gives the reader actual cases in both successful and less-than-successful attempts at establishing a parish nursing program.

With the specialty so new, this type of book provides the reader with a comprehensive array of information that is difficult to find in one source. It contains practical information about end-of-life issues, program evaluation, resource development, and much more. Also included are actual examples of forms and tools for the parish nurse to use in day-to-day practice. This is a book every parish nurse should have."

Cynthia R. Crabtree, EdD, MSN, RN
Dean, School of Nursing,
Spalding University,
Louisville, KY

This informative book will provide practical guidelines for nurses currrently in parish positions or those aspiring toward this helping role. The field needs dedicated professionals with a clear view of the problem of providing community service within the served community centered around faith establishments. This book provides helpful program development information from assessment to outcomes measurement.

Through personal case stories, practical ideas from past programs, and program outline samples, the professional is lead through the continuum of choice of parish nursing as a career to how to function within various faith health care services. This publication will assist the parish nurse in developing strategies for education, community programs, and funding to enable this faith and service nursing role to flourish."

Linda S. Dune, PhD, RN, CCRN, CEN
Assistant Professor of Clinical Nursing,
School of Nursing, Health Science Center,
University of Texas, Houston

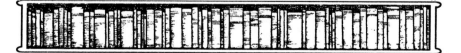

More pre-publication
REVIEWS, COMMENTARIES, EVALUATIONS . . .

"This book is a must for anyone interested in parish nursing. I only wish I could have read such a book to guide and inform me when I became interested in the field. This book is enlightening and highly educational. I predict it will become a foundational textbook that will be utilized by both schools of nursing and parish nursing organizations and others worldwide who have an interest in a health ministry."

Janet Quillian, DrPH, ARNP
Director of International Development Internship Program, Seattle University; Chairperson, St.James Cathedral Health and Healing Ministry, Seattle, WA

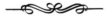

"A valuable characteristic of this book is its historical value. In years to come, it will be described as an intriguing and informative commentary on the continuing emergence of parish nursing as a specialty profession. Those who study the nature and development of professions will see in this work a classic redefinition of an existing profession (nursing) in response to changing health care issues and needs. The creative struggles to initiate and sustain parish nursing programs, the visionary efforts to combine nursing and pastoral care/counseling, and the clear identification of resources essential for the success of parish nursing, are set forth in first-person claims and confessions.

Further, this book highlights care of the aging and care at the end of life as two critical areas in health care that are currently problem-ridden and to which parish nursing, in the context of churches, may be an excellent response. It is an important addition to a field of health care and ministry striving for relevance and standing in today's world."

James L. Travis III, PhD
Director, Pastoral Services, Clinical Professor of Pastoral Care, Duke University Medical Center and Divinity School

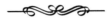

"Sybil Smith and the other contributors to this book have performed a valuable service to anyone interested in the parish nurse movement. The book carefully reviews the birth and evolution of parish nurse ministry. Descriptions of parish nurse programs provide helpful insights into considerations that may affect the ultimate success or dissolution of the programs. The testimonies of parish nurses give life to the struggles that too frequently attend the start of a new ministry or complicate its development, as well as the joys that can accompany the ministry. There is much of practical benefit in this book that would strengthen an existing parish nurse ministry or help those about to initiate a program avoid fatal or needless mistakes. This is a 'must-read' that provides mature perspective, practical guidance, theological insight, and a challenge to ministry that will inform parish nursing as it fulfills its vision to be an important component of the health ministry of the church."

Rev. Earl E. Shelp, PhD
President, Interfaith Care Partners, Houston, TX

Parish Nursing
A Handbook
for the New Millennium

THE HAWORTH PASTORAL PRESS
Religion and Mental Health
Harold G. Koenig, MD
Senior Editor

Parish Nursing
A Handbook
for the New Millennium

Sybil D. Smith, PhD, RN
Editor

The Haworth Pastoral Press®
An Imprint of The Haworth Press, Inc.
New York • London • Oxford

Published by

The Haworth Pastoral Press®, an imprint of The Haworth Press, Inc., 10 Alice Street, Binghamton, NY 13904-1580.

TR: 1.7.04

Cover design by Brooke Stiles.

Cover illustration of flower by Sister Marilyn Trowbridge.

Library of Congress Cataloging-in-Publication Data

Parish nursing : a handbook for the new millennium / Sybil D. Smith, editor.
    p.   ; cm.
Includes bibliographical references and index.
    ISBN 0-7890-1817-9 (hardcover : alk paper)—ISBN 0-7890-1818-7 (softcover : alk. paper)
  1. Parish nursing—Handbooks, manuals, etc.
    [DNLM: 1. Nursing—Handbooks. 2. Pastoral Care—Handbooks. 3. Religion—Handbooks. WY 49 P233 2003] I. Smith, Sybil D.
    RT120.P37 P368 2003
    610.73'43—dc21
                                          2002012076

This book is dedicated to my husband of thirty-nine years,
Michael Duane Smith.
Michael has been my best friend, a loyal critic,
and a faithful teacher.

CONTENTS

PART IV: PARISH NURSING AND END-OF-LIFE ISSUES

ABOUT THE EDITOR

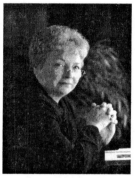 **Sybil D. Smith, PhD,** is Professor of Applied Gerontology at North Greenville College, Tigerville, South Carolina, where she developed a bachelor's degree program in that field from the mission/ministry model she used in parish nurse education. Dr. Smith has more than 30 years experience in community health and her classes on Health, Healing, and Wholeness© represent a mission/ministry model that emerged from her practice. She was affiliated with one of the largest volunteer parish nurse networks in the southeastern United States as an advisor and consultant, and later as an education specialist and coordinator, and has developed training modules for nurses transitioning from a hospital environment to community-based work.

Foreword

Parish nursing is growing like no other health care specialty. It was only about ten years ago, in 1992, that the first article on parish nursing appeared in Medline[1] (Medline database archives articles published since 1966). The first article in the Cumulative Index to Nursing and Allied Health appeared only one year earlier[2] (CINAHL database archives articles published since 1982). Despite the newness of this specialty, an estimated 3,000 parish nurses were employed throughout the United States by 1996.[3] Five years later, there were over 6,000.[4] Parish nursing, I believe, is the key to our ailing health care system today and most certainly in the years ahead.

In 2001, there were approximately 35 million people in the United States over the age of sixty-five. That number will remain relatively constant over the next five years, and then will start increasing rapidly around 2011 as 80 million baby boomers start turning age sixty-five. According to middle series estimates, over 77 million Americans will be over the age of sixty-five in the year in 2040.[5] If high series estimates are used, which are actually more likely given the impact new advances in research are having on longevity after age sixty-five, the number of persons age sixty-five or older in 2040 may approach 100 million. The growing elderly population is even more of an issue outside of the United States. Compared to other developed countries around the world, the United States is ranked thirty-third in terms of its aging population. By the year 2050, the United Nations has estimated that between 40 and 45 percent of the entire population of many countries in Europe will be over the age of sixty (38 percent for Japan and 33 percent for Russia).[6] Within the same time frame the support ratio (number of workers age eighteen to sixty-four divided by number of persons age sixty-five or older) is expected to drop from its current value of 5:1 down to 2:1 in developed countries throughout the world.

Even with only 35 million persons age sixty-five or over in the United States today, our health care system is already feeling the strain. The situation now, however, is likely to be the "best of times." The Medicare budget in 1965 was less than $5 billion per year; by 1980 it had increased to $38 billion and by 1992 to $135 billion. In 2000, total Medicare payments exceeded $238 billion.[7] By 2007, they are expected to rise above $415 billion.[8] Even now, many physicians are starting to refuse Medicare patients because payments are too low and are expected to drop even further; the American Academy of Family Physicians says that 17 percent of family doctors are not taking new Medicare patients.[9] If these problems are happening today, what will things look like in twenty to thirty years when the aging population doubles? Ed Schneider, Dean of the Leonard Davis School of Gerontology at the Andrus Gerontology Center (University of Southern California at Los Angeles), writing in the journal *Science,* estimates that in the year 2040 many older adults in the United States may be spending their later years without health care and living in city parks and on city streets.[10] He speculates that hospitals will accept only the sickest patients (and will resemble today's intensive care units) and then discharge them to nursing homes (which will resemble today's acute care hospitals). All other health care will back up into the community into people's homes. No longer will families be able to place their aging parents in nursing homes; such homes will simply be too full and waiting lists will be intolerably long. The pressure on families and society will be enormous, and many will seek relief in churches, synagogues, and temples.

What bothers me is that many parish nurses today have to go to great lengths to convince ministers, church boards, and congregations that having a health ministry is a worthy endeavor. Even when a parish nurse offers to volunteer for such a task, she or he often meets with resistance. However, given the demographic and economic trends just described, I am absolutely certain that parish nurses in future years will no longer have to beg their congregations to play a role in this area. As churches overflow with those who are sick, disabled, and chronically ill (and with the young families trying to care for the health needs of aging loved ones), I think all of this will change. Churches and congregations will be begging parish nurses to start health ministries to ease the burden on clergy that the huge demand for health care will create. Indeed, as throughout history, it was the church that came to the rescue of people experiencing poverty, sickness, and suffering. If the church does not assume this role again in the years ahead, I believe such a lack of response will foretell a decline in the role of the church in modern society.

Sybil Smith, who has been deeply immersed in health ministries for a decade, has brought together the writings of parish nurses in a way that gives an extraordinarily clear overview of parish nursing and an understanding of what the specialty is all about. This book will set the standard for an emerging field that offers hope and vision for not only our health care system but for all of those who are sick, for the religious congregations in which they worship, and for the profession of nursing itself. Nurses have become disillusioned as the profession has become more technologically focused—less a "calling" and more simply a job. Returning a spiritual focus to nursing is necessary and long overdue.

Harold G. Koenig, RN, MD
Associate Professor of Psychiatry and Medicine
Duke University Medical Center

NOTES

1. Margaret Drummond, Terry F. Buss, and Mary Ann Ladigo. "Volunteers for Community Health: An Ohio Hospital Sponsors Parish Nursing Programs for Area Churches and Synagogues," *Health Progress,* 73(5); 1992: 20-24.

2. Ann Solari-Twadell, "New Names, New Faces, and New Format," *Perspectives in Parish Nursing Practice,* 1(1); 1991: 1-2.

3. Jane A. Simington, Joanne K. Olson, and Lillian Douglass. "Promoting Well Being Within a Parish," *The Canadian Nurse,* 92; 1996: 20-24.

4. <http://www.marquette.edu/dept/nursing/parish.html>.

5. <http://www.aoa.gov/aoa/stats/AgePop2050.html>.

6. United Nations, *Population Aging—1999,* publication ST/ESA/SER.A/179 (United Nations, Population Division, Department of Economic and Social Affairs, 1999).

7. <http://www.seniors.gov/articles/0102/2000-health-costs.htm>.

8. Sheila Smith, Mark Freeland, Stephen Heffler, David McKusick, and The Health Expenditures Projection Team, "The Next Ten Years of Health Spending: What Does the Future Hold?" *Health Affairs,* 17; 1998: 128-140.

9. <http://senrs.com/many_doctors_say_they_are_refusing_medicare_patients.htm>.

10. Edward L. Schneider, "Aging in the Third Millennium," *Science,* 283; 1999: 796-797.

Preface

This text is a basic handbook with resources for starting and sustaining parish nurse ministry in the new millennium. It offers a framework that explains various approaches to parish nursing. For the first time, nurses and church leaders have a guide from which to design and structure a parish nursing program that complements the overall ministry goals of the congregation. The methods described in *Parish Nursing: A Handbook for the New Millennium* are derived from the fields of practice as lived out by committed nurses. I want to express my deep gratitude to all the contributors and thank them for their time commitment to the project.

I wish to acknowledge *Insights,* the Faculty Journal of Austin Presbyterian Theological Seminary, which first published my developing thoughts on the different approaches to parish nursing and graciously allowed me to include those thoughts in this work. I am indebted to Vicki Hollon, Executive Director of the Wayne E. Oates Institute, and Chris Hammon, Editor of *The Oates Journal,* both of whom encouraged me to further creativity and have granted permission for me to use materials they originally published in 2000. The work of Dr. Daniel Fountain has been a significant resource to me as an educator on the subject of the integration of faith and health, and I want to acknowledge the Billy Graham Center at Wheaton College and the William Cary Library for granting permission to reprint figures originally used by Dan Fountain and Lloyd Kwast, respectively.

Sister Marilyn Trowbridge, as a Franciscan Sister of the Poor, introduced parish nursing to South Carolina in the early 1990s. She did not have the availability of presentation resources as we do today. Most of her early presentations about parish nursing were given with visuals she personally created in a calligraphy-style art form. She donated drawings, originally prepared in 1994, for use in this book and they are inserted throughout the chapters. When I asked her about including a bio and photo, her remarks were, "I am not interested in the bio and photo. . . . To God be the Glory . . . after all, God deserves major credit. . . ." Many will remember one of her themes: "What you receive as a gift, give as a gift."

Introduction

Parish Nursing: A Handbook for the New Millennium is written by a complement of parish nurses and a health administrator, all of whom view parish nursing as ministry. The book is about the various gifts of ministry that each writer offers in stewardship of his or her faith. Not all contributors have the same spiritual gifts and talents, but they share a common mission. As pioneers in parish nurse ministry they serve with ministry gifts of administration, leadership, teaching, knowledge, wisdom, discernment, faith, help, mercy, giving, and healing. The contribution of each writer adds to improving the structural foundation for parish nursing of the future.

It is important to take a critical look at the past fifteen years in relation to the development of parish nursing in the United States. The purpose for looking back is to evaluate where we have been and to gain insight on how to go forward. Parish nursing in the new millennium will be different from parish nursing of the past decade. The future for parish nursing is challenged by growing numbers of elderly and shrinking health care resources. Because of the shift in demography, dollars, and the health care workforce, this book does not address the whole of parish nursing. The assumption is that the rising number of elderly will encourage congregations to support parish nurse ministries to the aging, whereas in the past a congregation may not have been interested in paying a nurse for generalist type health promotion activities.

Few denominations had executive level support for parish nursing in the early 1990s. Solid foundational structure for parish nursing, in the example of executive-level decisions to promote parish nursing from denominational headquarters in the Lutheran Church Missouri Synod, is noted. Many congregations first learned about parish nursing through methodology described in Chapter 3 by Dr. Renae Schumann. Dr. Schumann's story demonstrates the entrepreneurial spirit of commitment and creativity necessary in times of emerging structure.

The emerging structure for parish nursing of the 1990s is in the context of the failure of health care reform. Health care futurists and planners had ideas and agendas that parish nurses watched come and go. As parish nurses affiliated with hospitals watched these agendas come and go, some also saw their positions come and go. In the backdrop of health care politics were the struggles within parish nursing groups regarding professional organizational support of the new parish nursing subspecialty. Little of the parish nurse education of the past decade was anchored to schools and colleges of nursing. It is difficult to understand the issues about parish nurse education without first exploring the larger picture of nursing education in general.

The "whatever works" or pragmatic program development approaches of the 1990s created two areas of frustration. The first was related to the sluggishness in assessing where parish nursing fit into the larger picture of health, organizations, and politics. This first area of frustration drove the second area of frustration: weak program evaluation methods. Understanding the motivations behind parish nurse programs is essential in addressing parish nursing within the bigger view of organizations and politics. It was easier for denomination-based parish nurse programs to match the mission, goals, and values of their anchor organizations. Parish nurse programs based in secular hospitals became involved with congregations by entering into individualized agreements or contracts with each particular congregation. In these agreements or contract situations program evaluation was complex because there were multiple constituents to satisfy.

As an integral part of communities of faith, parish nurses of the future will be confronted with end-of-life issues as congregations become more involved in ministries to the aging. Nurses need an academic understanding of end-of-life issues. Parish nurses of the future will be confronted to reevaluate the *Scope and Standards of Parish Nursing Practice* in light of the appropriateness for parish nurses to be more than referral agents and listeners when working with families and individuals dealing with end of life. The question is asked, in light of health care workforce issues, about the suitability of parish nurses engaging the concepts of hospice and palliative care.

As a society we cannot yet visualize the needs of individuals, families, and congregations in the new millennium as they relate to aging issues. We can talk about the age wave coming; when we do, it is in terms of the current frame of reference of hospitals, nursing homes, filial caregivers, and social service networks. We often speak of the rising number of elderly, without making the connection to resource allocation and health workforce issues. The health care structure that surrounds us today cannot make the stretch for the demands ahead. Euthanasia and assisted suicide concerns will surface along with other end-of-life issues. End-of-life issues represent appropriate themes for congregational involvement from two levels. First is the spiritual care and support needed by those involved in such difficult decision making. Second is the direct provision by congregations of care for the dying. The current political climate is pressed with issues related to euthanasia and physician-assisted suicide. These issues will challenge congregations of the future to engage the bioethics arena and confront their values on the sanctity and dignity of human life. Parish nurses are appropriate additions to ministry staffs for the management of ministries to the aging and dying.

PART I:
PLANNING FOR NEW MILLENNIUM PARISH NURSING

Chapter 1

A New Landscape for Parish Nursing

Sybil D. Smith

Various ministry opportunities are emerging for churches in relation to the current discourse on health, healing, and wholeness in and among communities of faith. Ministries in nursing are considered such an opportunity. Many terms are related to health programs in local churches, such as *parish nursing, congregational nursing, health ministries,* and *church-based health promotion,* to name a few. The varying terms used to describe ministries of health can be confusing and cloud underlying philosophies that may be difficult to distinguish in the beginning. The purpose of this text is to offer a clearer lens through which to view nursing programs in churches, and to provide a basic handbook with resources for the practice of parish nursing in the new millennium. A new landscape for parish nurses is being painted. This text will bridge the Westberg era of parish nursing to the next stage of expansion with the goal of contributing to the development of solid structures for parish nursing programs.

Accomplishments during the Westberg era include awakening the hearts of nurses to nearly forgotten traditions, calling communities of faith to be accountable for whole-person health, raising to consciousness the term *parish nursing,* describing roles for parish nurses, and developing the International Parish Nurse Resource Center (IPNRC). The IPNRC advanced the parish nursing concept by developing educational opportunities and hosting the annual Westberg Symposium, a network gathering for hundreds of parish nurses. During the Westberg era, the Health Ministries Association was formed as a membership organization and was recognized by the American Nurses Association as the voice for parish nurses. In 1998, the *Scope and Standards of Parish Nursing Practice* was published jointly by the Health Ministries Association and the American Nurses Association.[1]

In bridging the Westberg era of parish nursing to the new millennium, two matters are relevant. First, the new millennium itself invites a retrospective and prospective assessment of the state of the knowledge, utility, and direction of parish nursing. Second, the change of ownership announced October 19, 2001, of the IPNRC from the Lutheran-rooted Advocate Health Care System to the Deaconess Foundation of St. Louis, Missouri, was unexpected news. Both of these matters in light of a post–September 11, 2001, reality paint a new landscape for parish nursing. This chapter describes the new landscape for parish nursing, introduces the new leadership of the International Parish Nurse Resource Center, addresses structural integrity, reflects on the past decade, and envisions new foundations for parish nurse programs.

THE NEW LANDSCAPE

In his classic, *The Wounded Healer,* Henri Nouwen related that God calls His people to recognize the suffering of their time, as well as to become responsive.[2] The turn of a century is certainly an appropriate time to reflect critically on the past and evaluate the potential of the future. With respect to those who feel one cannot let demography become destiny, the fact remains that demography is a tool of science that allows us to chart future needs. In looking to the future, several scenes emerge. The emerging demographic landscape represents a potential for much suffering in the lives of individuals, families, and communities as they face the needs of the elderly. Caring for the older population will have consequences for all strata. Not only will older persons be at risk for lack of services and resource allocation issues, but the burden of caregiving will become ever present in the lives of family members and communities of faith. Parish nurses of the new millennium will be on the front lines of these issues surrounding older Americans and their family members.

The Rising Number of Elderly

The rising number of older Americans is dramatic. The world, including the United States, is "graying." There are over 34 million people in the United States over age sixty-five, which constitutes

13 percent of the total U.S. population. This number will rise to 20 percent of the U.S. population by the year 2030. The highest growth rate in the United States is for the over-eighty-five population and there are an increasing number of centenarians. Increases in the older age groups are due to increases in life expectancy, which rose to 76.5 in 1997. The number of minorities in the over-sixty-five population will rise from 13 to 25 percent by the year 2030. The largest increases in minorities will be for Asians and Pacific Islanders, followed by Hispanics and non-Hispanic blacks.[3] The rising number of elderly has considerable implications for parish nursing from both obvious and not-so-obvious perspectives.

An obvious consideration explores just who will take care of so many older persons. The children of the over-eighty-five group may themselves be impaired from chronic disease and aging processes, and therefore, unable to care for a parent. For various reasons, some adult children may feel no filial responsibility for aging parents. A very mobile society of the past few decades has many adult children living at distances from their parents. A 1998 study by The National Alliance for Caregiving addresses the phenomenon of caregiving in the United States.[4] The statistics provide a picture of the typical caregiver:

- Women account for 73 percent of caregivers.
- The average caregiver is forty-six years old.
- Thirty-nine percent of caregivers are between the ages of thirty-five and forty-nine years.
- Sixty-six percent of caregivers are married.
- Half of all caregivers are employed full-time; 12 percent are part-time workers.
- The median income of caregivers' households is $35,000.

For adult children who assume the care of parents, many stresses and strains can develop. Not only will there be physical demands of caring for the older parent, but all family members will be impacted. For instance, an adult child caring for a bedridden parent will not be available to attend all of the school functions of his or her own children or grandchildren. Fatigue and burnout are common among caregivers, with high rates of physical illness and depression reported, as well as loss of employment and subsequent loss of income over time.[5] Congregations will be expected to provide support and ministries as their members cope with issues of aging parents and late-life transitions.

A less obvious perspective is the societal consequence we are living out: widespread public denial concerning long-term care risk.[6] Many do not prepare for long-term care. They wait until a crisis occurs. Parish nurses may have to stretch to create health promotion programs for families caring for older persons. Transportation needs, adaptive equipment needs, and respite care needs, when left unmet, can place older persons at risk as well as add to the burden of those responsible for their care. Out of necessity, parish nurses of the future are likely to become coordinators of services for the elderly. Congregations can contribute to meeting the long-term care needs of the community. A question to grapple with is, Should a congregation provide aging ministries to members only or make it available to all within a geographic boundary of the church?

Redefining Long-Term Care

Because of the rising number of elderly, a second scene is projected on the landscape of the new millennium in the form of increased demands for home care, hospice, palliative, and community-based services. Health care workers understand that the continuum of long-term care includes both community- and institution-based services, but church members may lack adequate knowledge about the options available and how they are accessed. The Medicaid system, allowing for sheltering of assets, has generated entitlement thinking among even the prosperous who can manipulate assets, qualify for Medicaid, and enter nursing homes without tapping the equity in their home.[7] The current long-term care system will be redefined as resources become scarce and increased numbers of older Americans will be cared for within the community. Caring congregations will be challenged to respond to the demand, and perhaps strained to provide support at both a theological and sociological level.

From a theological perspective, those in situations of pain, suffering, and disability will look to caring communities of faith to find meaning and purpose in their suffering. As a death-denying society, we are not prepared as individuals to live with a long course of declining health and loss of functioning abilities. Those who care for suffering persons will also seek answers. From a sociological dimension of aging, communities of faith in true fellowship provide an opportunity to share one another's burden. Sharing in one another's suffering requires a mature faith by those who participate in the caregiving. A strong faith is also required of the recipients of care as they grow in the ministry of dependence.[8]

Learning the ministry of dependence will be a challenge. Do older persons want to be old in our dependence-fearing culture? If autonomy and self-sufficiency are seen as virtue in the prime of vocational careers, just how does one learn to set aside such virtue and become a dependent recipient of care? Mary Pipher relates that the expectation of aging parents needing their children has become a shameful secret, and that the change in the meaning of the word *dependency* to signify something shameful is resultant of our therapized culture.[9] The later life struggle with dependency is a spiritual issue and appropriately addressed within the community of faith.

End-of-Life Issues and Resource Allocation

The demands for increased community and home care services bring about a third scene on the landscape of the new century, resource allocation. Resource allocation differs somewhat in shape from unequal access to health care issues. Resource allocation is the logical extension of the access to health care issues that went unresolved in the 1990s, and opens a discourse on bioethics and end-of-life issues. According to John Kilner, resource allocation will raise questions about who should live when not all can live, and just who will receive donated organs.[10] Will age become the criteria for scarce resources? Kilner further relates that important distinctions will have to be considered between terminal versus imminent; withdrawing versus withholding treatment; relieving pain versus ending life; and extraordinary care versus burdensome care. Are congregations currently staffed with persons gifted and talented enough to walk alongside families facing such dilemmas?

In the 1990s, many community collaborations delved into sponsorship of parish nurse initiatives and brought to the forefront an awareness of the inequities of the U.S. health care system. All of the identified justifications for parish nurse programs of the 1990s still exist and will be compounded over the next several decades by the rising number of elderly, the increased demand for community-based services, and the confrontation between resource allocation and end-of-life issues.

Communities of faith have been slow to respond to bioethics in aging issues. Resource allocation and end-of-life issues will cause families to seek out communities of faith for assistance in ways they perhaps have not in the past. In sensitivity and responsiveness to potential sufferings of the new millennium, sustaining structures within congregations will have to be erected to support parish nurse ministries. Since the early 1990s parish nurses have looked to the annual conference known as the Westberg Symposium, sponsored by the IPNRC, for guidance and updates on trends in parish nursing. The IPNRC focused on an education curriculum while structure was allowed to emerge. With anticipation, parish nurses are looking to the new leadership of IPNRC for new millennium direction.

A WORD FROM THE NEW EXECUTIVE DIRECTOR OF THE IPNRC

Rev. Deborah Patterson

Everywhere you turn today you find a plethora of health information, from the cover of *Time* magazine to the brochure racks at grocery stores. Add television and the Internet, and there is no shortage of health information before the eyes of the public. Then add the most up-to-date health care technology for diagnostic and treatment interventions, from CT scans to lasers and beyond. To that add our nation's health care professionals and those who work with them—doctors, nurses, social workers, occupational therapists, physical therapists, and others. Finally, pour on a healthy dose of spending—over 16 percent of the U.S. gross domestic product at the time of this writing—and you have a recipe for a healthy nation. Or do you?

Substance abuse, alcohol abuse, and domestic violence are rampant. Loneliness is a complaint heard obliquely, if not directly, by health professionals every day. In fact, loneliness has been called the number-one

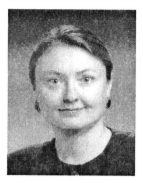

Reverend Deborah Patterson, an ordained United Church of Christ clergywoman, is Executive Director of the International Parish Nurse Resource Center/Deaconess Parish Nurse Ministries in St. Louis. Prior to her work at the IPNRC/DPNM, she was Vice President of the Deaconess Foundation, a health foundation in St. Louis that supports parish nursing and children's health initiatives in the St. Louis metropolitan area, and she also served as a local pastor for several years. She is a graduate of Eden Theological Seminary and holds a master's degree in health administration from Washington University in St. Louis.

killer in America today. We are overweight, overstressed, and out of shape. With all of that health information and technology available today, what is going on?

The average American life expectancy has increased by more than thirty years since the turn of the twentieth century to 76.5 years today, but most of that increase can be attributed to improvements in public health—cleaner food, air, and water, and changes in lifestyle—not to medical technologies or drugs. Therefore it would seem relatively important to support public health initiatives. Yet few of our health-related dollars in this country are spent on public health. The church is a place where public health initiatives can thrive, for a minimal cost.

The church, at the forefront of health care in the 1800s, became intimidated by technology and its dazzle and price tags, and took a backseat in the mid-twentieth century, abrogating its leadership role in healing. The parish nurse program is a return to the roots of nursing practice as it was envisioned in the middle of the nineteenth century, while supporting the best of the current health care climate. The first nurses were deeply inspired by their spiritual beliefs regarding healing and acted on those impulses. They also acted based on good science, which was not seen as separate from acting in faithful response to God's call. Public health measures, such as hand washing promoted by Florence Nightingale and other early nurses, were responsible for huge increases in survival rates by patients. These early nurses cared for body and soul.

The church should be appalled that over 40 million Americans have no health insurance. Parish nurses are speaking out on this subject. The church should be distressed that nearly 100,000 people per year die as a result of accidental injuries caused by medical treatment. Parish nurses are aware of this and serve as advocates to those working their way through the health care system. The church should be strongly recommending healthy lifestyles full of exercise and proper nutrition. Parish nurses are promoting wellness, and doing much, much more.

Parish nurses understand the school of thought being demonstrated by the recently released Harvard Study of Adult Development, currently directed by George E. Vaillant, MD, which studied health and sociological data on the lives of Harvard graduates over a course of more than fifty years. This study, published as a book by Dr. Vaillant under the title *Aging Well,* demonstrates that a strong social network, a loving marriage, and a positive attitude, combined with good health habits, create a person more likely to age well than someone without these strengths. These are strengths that a congregation can nurture.[11]

Parish nurses also know that in our mobile society, there is often no one to take care of aging adults. They know that as more women work outside the home, they have fewer hours free for volunteer caregiving to the homebound and others needing help. They know that the health care system is complicated, and that people can fall through the cracks. They know many people are intimidated by physicians and afraid to speak up for themselves, or may not understand the implications of a diagnosis or treatment.

Parish nurses, to quote one with whom I work, "have no length of stay." They can work with individuals within a family system, within a congregational system, and within a community. They can work with that person, that family, that congregation, for years. Most, in fact, do just that. The turnover rate among parish nurses is very low. The satisfaction rate among parish nurses is very high.

Most parish nurses take their role as integrators of faith and health very seriously. They have spent years working as nurses in other capacities before coming to parish nursing, developing their skills and strengths. They know that all healing is miraculous and comes in three ways: through the natural healing of the body; through assistance to help the body heal; or through death, which is a natural part of life. In all these ways, parish nurses work to keep parishioners with health concerns (and that is all parishioners, at some point) in close community with others, and in close contact with God, the healer of the nations. In addition, most parish nurses reach out beyond the congregation to serve others in need as well.

At this time in our history, when our planet seems so vulnerable, with war in many lands, even attacks here on our own soil, the healing presence of the Church is needed more than ever. Parish nursing is moving from primarily a Christian ministry to a nursing practice within other faiths as well. We were saddened by the closing of the International Parish Nurse Resource Center in Chicago, but cheered at the prospect of continuing the legacy set forth over the past fifteen years by continuing the Westberg Symposium and participating in updating the Parish Nurse Basic Preparation Curriculum, in partnership with so many wonderful parish nurse programs that have developed over the years.

Parish nursing exists now in many different models, both paid and volunteer, part time and full time, as part of a network or striking out on one's own. There are probably close to 5,000 parish nurses in the United States at this time, and parish nurses are growing in number in other countries as well. The local program with which I am affiliated in St. Louis is Deaconess Parish Nurse Ministries. We will also continue the work of the International Parish Nurse Resource Center from St. Louis, under the IPNRC name. For more information about our programs, please visit our Web site at <www.parishnurses.org> or call us at (314) 918-2559.

To all that work in parish nursing and support its ministry and practice, we say, "Blessings! The time is ripe, and the need is great." Or as Jesus would say, "The fields are white unto harvest." We are into the third millennium since Jesus' birth, but we need parish nursing and a return to caring for one another in faith communities and our surrounding communities now more than ever.

STRUCTURAL INTEGRITY

The structure of a parish nursing program is the arrangement of the interrelated components necessary to deliver parish nurse ministry. Are the interrelated components available, and are they reliable enough to support the demands of effective parish nurse ministry?

In the past, organizational structures were ill suited for parish nurse programs for several reasons. First, parish nursing was new and people had to warm to the concept. The concept of parish nursing was accepted slowly in local churches often because it was not understood at the denominational headquarters level, which prevented hierarchical encouragement to the local congregations. Second, many parish nurse programs of the 1990s were launched on grant or soft monies, and program evaluation methods were often unable to provide the necessary data to continue soft monies or permanent sources of funding. Third, parish nurses themselves were solidifying their own identity. Supporting structures at several levels need to be created for parish nurse programs of the future. At the disciplinary level, issues about parish nurse education and certification need to be clarified. The new ownership of the IPNRC may be able to bring consensus to the varying contingencies among those who practice parish nursing. Local congregational structures can become stronger when ecclesiastical and denominational headquarters support parish nursing. With support from denominational headquarters, the local churches can address more seriously the administrative structure needed for delivery of parish nurse ministry. At the personal level, parish nurses must commit to professional accountability as well as spiritual growth and development.

As the new millennium is embraced, a growing comfort with the concept of parish nursing is evidenced by the number of educational programs available. Parish nurse education is addressed today with vocational programs of core curriculum, school of nursing courses, and graduate programs. The 1998 publication of the *Scope and Standards of Parish Nursing Practice* strengthened the identity of parish nursing as a subspecialty in nursing. However, few congregations take full responsibility and pay a parish nurse as a staff member. Soft monies are not the answer for developing a solid foundation from which viable parish nurse ministries can flourish and meet the challenges of an aging population.

LESSONS IN REFLECTION

At the time of this writing thirteen mainline denominations were listed on the Health Ministries Association (HMA) Web site <www.

healthministriesassociation.org> as denominational chapters of HMA. An informal telephone and e-mail survey to the contact person cited for each of the denominational chapters was conducted. The following questions were asked:

1. How many volunteer parish nurses do you have who volunteer one day per week or more, and how many volunteer less than one day per week?
2. How many parish nurses do you have who are paid by the congregation in which they serve and what is the average number of hours worked? Are they considered church staff and have a benefit package?
3. How many parish nurses do you have who are paid by outside funding sources such as grants, hospitals, and collaborative community efforts?
4. Does your parish nurse programming target church members only, all persons within a radius of the church, or a deprived segment of the population such as a housing project, underprivileged area church, or the developmentally challenged, to name a few?
5. Are you a registered nurse and are you paid by denominational headquarters?

Two of the denominational chapter contact persons responded saying they had received the survey, did not have the data, but would forward the request "up the line" and named the office to which the request was sent. Another reported that the chapter did not keep that data but did have a Web site where parish nursing was recognized and the names and locations of the parish nurses were listed. Three responded relating they had a mix of volunteers and soft-money-paid nurses, and two of these had denominational Web site support for parish nurse ministry. Only one reported with an exact number of 241 parish nurses within their denomination, Web site coverage, and a part-time, paid, denominational coordinator who worked under a Program Minister of Health and Wellness. There was no response from six of the denominational chapter contact people. Generalizations cannot be made from these types of data but questions can be asked about the essence of parish nursing within these organizations. Perhaps the biggest accomplishment in the 1990s was establishing the concept and presence of parish nursing; the challenge for developing sustaining structure lies ahead.

Social Accountability

In the 1990s many health systems and hospitals responded to social accountability pressures with support for parish nurse programs. Parish nurse programs were a way for hospitals to demonstrate to the community a concern for establishing a safety net for those without health insurance. Health system resources were often coupled with private foundation resources and partnerships developed with congregations for various motivations.[12] Community health needs and current resources were assessed. Whether or not systems of care were impacted by these efforts is unclear. When the supporting denominations of parish nurse programs are not sure today of just how many parish nurses they have, paid or unpaid, one can assume program evaluation methods have not been a priority.

Many of the large start-up grants awarded for parish nurse programs were for three-year periods. Perhaps in a rush to implement and deliver results in a three-year time frame, program planners overlooked reliable organizational planning frameworks. In defense of early planners, one must be mindful of the postmodern philosophies of the 1990s. Soft boundaries abounded. Relativistic thinkers touted emerging structure, moaned the profit motive in health care, and cried for equal access to health care. Idealistic and naive people failed to recognize that profits were made in health care long before the emergence of private for-profit entities. In ethical situations associated with revenue generation, including the capitalist extreme of profiteering, personal values may not be congruent with what is legal and expected in American society.[13] Health care in the United States is political and reform did not happen as anticipated in the 1990s.

Ann Solari-Twadell presents a three-year time line for development of a parish nurse program, recommending the selection and hiring of a nurse take place in year two.[14] Many of the start-up grants of the past decade did not allow enough time for development of solid structure. Hopefully a well-thought-out structure will contribute to serious endorsements for parish nursing in the future.

Denominational Support for Parish Nursing

In a denomination where support for parish nursing is obvious, such as Web site recognition, individuals hearing about the parish nurse concept for the first time have a point of reference that is nonthreatening. The journey is difficult for nurses heeding a spiritual call to parish nurse ministries when there is no denominational support. When the nurse speaks of parish nursing to the pastor or other church members and there is no reference point supporting parish nursing within the denomination, it can take a very long time to implement a program. Contrasting reflections will be presented in two personal accounts. Koby's story is one of denominational support and Nadine's story takes another course.

Koby's Story

My experience with parish nursing started in the fall of 1997. Our church was one of five churches in the area that was introduced to parish nursing through a grant sponsored by the Duke Endowment and Park Ridge Hospital of Fletcher, North Carolina. Our church, St. James Episcopal of Hendersonville, North Carolina, was offered a registered nurse who was paid by the grant for twenty hours a week. I knew very little at that time about what our parish nurse did because I never needed any of the services that she was able to provide or coordinate. The nurse completed the eighteen-month trial period offered by the grant, but left the position because the church was unable to take over the responsibility of providing her salary and benefits once the grant period ended.

In April 1999, I was feeling unfulfilled in my position as a public health nurse at our local health department. I prayed for guidance and

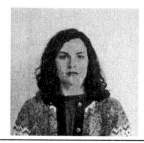

Koby MacFarland, RN, graduated from Rush University, Chicago, in 1991. Her work experiences include pediatric and neonatal intensive care, intravenous home therapy for oncology and HIV-positive children, public health, and parish nursing. She completed a distance-learning program in parish nursing from Concordia University in Alberta, Canada, directed by Dr. Lynda Miller.

some sign as to what I should be doing. One night in the middle of literally praying out loud in desperation, the words *parish nurse* were said to me in a voice other than my own. I peacefully fell asleep. The next morning I called our rector, Father Alex Viola, and told him how I was feeling and what had happened during the night. I asked if our church had any plans to continue the parish nurse program. He answered yes, and asked me to come speak with him. Although I knew nothing about what a parish nurse was or did, the Holy Spirit was guiding me, and I was at peace. I interviewed and within two weeks I became the new parish nurse at St. James.

Since our church was now solely responsible for employing the parish nurse, I started with ten hours a week and no benefits. I had two very small children at home and ten hours per week worked out well. However, I learned that ten hours a week was not enough time to carry out my duties. Early on I proposed to the vestry and the parish the need to increase the hours of the program.

As mentioned earlier, I knew very little about what a parish nurse did, and I quickly learned that much of our parish felt the same confusion. In September I enrolled in a distance-education course for basic parish nurse preparation through Concordia University in Alberta, Canada, to learn more about parish nursing. The program was financed by the church, took twelve weeks to complete, and was the most beneficial thing I did to prepare for my new role. I was encouraged that I could develop the parish nurse program into something that could touch many, not only in our parish but also in our whole community. In terms of networking and aiding my role as educator, I attended educational conferences when they were offered locally. A budget was set up for the program and I was allowed to use the funds at my discretion. To me, the freedom in the budget arrangement symbolized regard of the parish nurse as a professional. I was always expected to attend the Tuesday staff meetings.

The education gained from the parish nurse curriculum at Concordia helped me to establish policies specific to my church and my state's licensure requirements. I was able to format some documentation of my visitations and the programs offered. I became able to answer the questions about what a parish nurse does and why the church needs a parish nurse.

Encouragement for the program was reinforced by our clergy, the vestry, and mostly by those persons to whom I was able to provide visitation, coordinate services, and to the families of those who benefitted from the program. As a parish nurse, some of my responsibilities involved visitation, offering of Holy Eucharist to our homebound parishioners, and coordination of community services, including establishing emergency medical contact services such as Life Line. I did a full hands-on evaluation of sixteen of our local nursing and health care homes and retirement facilities to offer our parishioners a quick statistical review of what our county had to offer. We were able to provide programs to both educate and support the parishioners with health promotion and preventive health care seminars. I coordinated blood drives and even provided a program in which forty of our parishioners were able to get their health care power of attorney, advance directives, and living will paperwork in order, and were comforted in knowing that this often scary and dreaded process was complete.

Support of our program grew over time; in January 2001, the church was able to increase my pay to nineteen hours per week; still no benefits, but we were on our way. Our assistant rector, Father Robert Salamone, said once to our parish, "It is hard to really know what Koby does and how she helps those in our parish until or unless you have needed her. Her assets are those of presence, comfort, guidance, support, and education. If you haven't needed her, then you have been lucky. But if you have needed her, you know that what she and this program can offer you is invaluable." The nineteen hours certainly aided in meeting the demands of the ministry and the needs of our parishioners. The church acknowledged that this program needed a full-time registered nurse.

I left my position of parish nurse in May 2001 because of a personal need to be home with my three-and-a-half and five-and-a-half-year-old sons. The decision to leave my role was a difficult one, but the Holy Spirit brought me into parish nursing and the Holy Spirit told me to go home to my children. I knew that my time as parish nurse served not only to meet the needs of our parishioners, but to establish the structure for the program while making our parish aware of its significance. Parish nursing is as much about being a spiritual caregiver as it is about being an educator, liaison to the clergy, parishioner advocate, and coordinator of community services and health counselor. God was in everything I did as a parish nurse and He provided me with an extraordinary experience.

This story does not end in May 2001. In October, St. James Episcopal Church hired a new parish nurse and although the church is still only able to provide nineteen hours a week, the church continues the support of the ministry. I truly believe that as time goes on I will one day be able to make an addendum to this story and tell you that St. James has a full-time parish nurse. Until then, know that the parish nurse is critical in tying together all the aspects of health and putting God back into health care where He has always been and always belongs.

Nadine's Story

In fall 1995, I was approaching retirement and wondering how I would fill my time. One of the things I wanted to do was renew my fellowship with the Lord. Even though I was coteaching a Sunday school class, I no longer felt close to the Lord so I enrolled in a ten-week "Experiencing God" course at my church. In this course I confronted past issues in my life that had never been resolved. With God's help, I was able to resolve a forgiveness issue, truly experience God, and look for a way to serve Him.

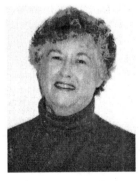

Nadine P. Bridwell, MN, CANP, RN, entered nursing practice as a diploma graduate and later completed a BSN and MN and successfully completed the certification exam to practice as a certified adult nurse practitioner. Nadine is a retired nurse educator with twenty years of teaching experience, eight of which were spent in the area of gerontology and end-of-life issues. She also served seven years as a nurse practitioner in a nursing home. While employed in the nursing home, Nadine noticed that persons with diabetes could receive foot care from a podiatrist that was Medicaid reimbursable. Persons without diabetes and other qualifying medical diagnoses received no foot care, only bathing. Driven by the deplorable condition of untended feet and nails, Nadine pursued special training in the care of feet and nails, which was carried forward in her parish nurse practice.

Since my strength is my nursing ability I approached one of our pastors about holding a foot clinic at our church. With the pastor's agreement and the help of another nurse in my church, the foot clinic was a success. A few weeks later I noticed a newspaper ad by the local Catholic hospital, encouraging nurses to come to a free workshop and learn about parish nursing. After attending the first class I knew God was calling me to parish nurse ministry. I shared my feelings with the senior pastor who was very enthusiastic and felt parish nursing would be a way the church could minister to the elderly members. The pastor advised me to prepare a short statement for the deacon board. I did, and the board approved the development of the parish nurse ministry under my guidance.

An office was provided. The parish nurse office opened officially on April 17, 1996. It was the first parish nurse program in our area. Another nurse, with a regular full-time job, helped and we held office hours on Wednesday afternoon (just before the midweek prayer service) for blood pressure screening, blood sugar screening, discussion, and questions related to health problems. In addition to these duties, the pastor sometimes called and asked me to visit certain members of the congregation who were either sick or were caring for someone they loved who was sick.

We promoted a screening for prostate cancer and breast cancer, and offered classes taught by various professionals who were members of our congregation. We developed an advisory committee that was, unfortunately, not helpful, so it was left to me to try to identify the health needs of the church. I sensed some tension among other health care workers in the church who worked for a health system other than the one I looked to for educational and resource support.

When the senior pastor relocated to another congregation, I received limited support from an associate pastor. During the interim, we held a health fair for adults and a safety fair for children. When our new senior pastor arrived, he was made aware of the parish nurse office and the services we performed. Although he is very favorable in his conversations, he does not refer members and leaves the decisions to us as to the kinds of duties we feel comfortable handling. We continue to open the office every Wednesday afternoon and often hold foot clinics. We write an article about health for the church newsletter once a month, and coordinate health screenings for various vascular problems.

It would be much easier if we had some direction from the pastoral staff. It would also be helpful if we were truly thought of as an extension of the ministerial staff. It is our feeling that because we are volunteer nurses we are not as valued as we would be if we were considered staff. Our denominational association of twenty-nine churches has only one other church interested in parish nursing even though they have all been informed about the benefits of parish nursing.

Observations

Koby's story of denominational level support is representative of what can happen when parish nurse ministry is valued in the hierarchal structure of a community of faith. Nadine's story reveals what one persistent nurse can accomplish over time; however, after six years, the administrative board of the church does not value the ministry enough to view a nurse as ministry staff. Many nurses in the 1990s were drawn to the concept of parish nursing but never saw it become a reality in their community of faith.

Volunteer Models of Parish Nursing

The volunteer approach to parish nurse ministries contributes very little to solid structure. The following are my personal observations while affiliated with a hospital-sponsored volunteer parish nurse network in the 1990s. The reflections are summarized and reprinted with permission.[15]

Three areas of concern surfaced: (1) church volunteers versus ministry staff, (2) pastoral and administrative support, and (3) professional accountability. Being a part of ministry staff denotes more responsibility than just another church volunteer. The term "ministry staff" denotes responsibilities and expectations from both the church and the nurse, whereas responsibility is somewhat negotiable when the term *volunteer* is used. The pastoral and administrative leadership need to give visible support for the nurse ministry and clearly identify the role of the parish nurse in the church's overall local mission. Even though the nurse experiences a "spiritual calling" to serve in his or her congregation, the "spiritual calling" does not negate responsibility to the public regulations that apply to the professional nurse who is licensed according to the Nurse Practice Act of the state in which they practice.

Can a nurse who works a full-time public job do justice on a volunteer basis to the position of ministry staff? Does a nurse who is retired want to do all that is required for professional accountability? From my observations of seventy volunteer nurses across ten counties in thirty-four congregations, I feel the volunteer model leaves much to be desired. In looking back, valuable lessons are learned and future direction can be charted. If September 11, 2001, began the closure of postmodernism, as some suggest, it will now be easier to go forward holding to tenets of developing solid structural foundations for parish nurse programs.

Nadine's story is one in which the emerging structure concept for a volunteer program offered little, but because she was retired and had the availability of time, she was able to persist. Competing hospitals in the 1990s sometimes touted parish nurse programs with one-upmanship and contributed to parish nurse turnoff in some denominations and geographic regions. The attempted advisory committee in Nadine's story was made up of mostly people from health care vocations who were employed by competing health systems.

REVISIONING THE FOUNDATION

Strong administrative support and endorsement within the congregation is needed to develop a solid foundation for parish nurse ministry. Structure is needed administratively for fiscal, philosophical, and theological identity. A clear definition of health and healing needs to be articulated and shared by administrative boards and the parish nurse. Various faith traditions define health and healing differently, based on the belief about the source of suffering and healing. Parish nurses must confront the terms of health and healing in a personal way that most likely was not taught in traditional nursing programs. Health and healing from solely a clinical picture is incomplete. Working definitions of health and healing for a parish nurse are personal and can fall on a continuum from an incomplete to a complete picture of *shalom wholeness* which draws forth peacefulness in the midst of suffering. Lynda Miller describes shalom wholeness as dwelling at peace and in harmony in all relationships: within oneself, with God, with other people, and with the created natural world.[16] In her nursing model grounded in Christian faith, Miller further explicates that personal shalom wholeness is possible only through a personal relationship with Christ. Understanding shalom wholeness is a growth process.

A conflict exists with what the health care marketplace implies about health and healing. In the marketplace, health care is a commodity driven by economic values promoting products such as instructional, surgical, and pharmacological interventions for physical well-being. Persons may not fully realize or search for the difference until a crisis comes into their lives. Many begin the journey of learning about their faith system's view of health and healing when a specific need develops. Health is more than the external guidelines for healthy lifestyle such as diet, exercise, and stress reduction. The desired outcome is the internal discovery processes that take place in the journey of faith which cause one to choose God's ways to health, healing, and wholeness.[17]

The journey of faith and discovery of the internal processes that can promote health and healing seem like a leap from the health care marketplace. In the United States confidence has been placed in doctors, medicine, and surgery for the promotion of health and healing. Even when we claim in humility that God guides the hands of those who render health care to us, it is an incomplete picture of health and healing. The substance of one's faith is called to bear on defining health and healing.

SUMMARY

In summary, the new landscape for parish nurse ministries includes responsiveness to the demands made by the rising numbers of elderly in light of resource allocation issues. This responsiveness will require structural integrity at the disciplinary, congregational, and individual levels. The postmodern softness of boundaries experienced in the 1990s will not provide the structure needed for future demands. Allowing structures to emerge in the past decade did get the concept of parish nursing launched, but lacked the form and shape needed for parish nursing in the new millennium. Within congregations, administrative restructuring for parish nurse ministry is needed.[18] A time-out is necessary to forge the structure that will bear the weight of future needs. Strategic planning for structure will be discussed in Chapter 6.

NOTES

1. Health Ministries Association, Inc. and American Nurses Association, *Scope and Standards of Parish Nursing Practice* (Washington, DC: American Nurses Publishing, 1998).

2. Henri Nouwen, introduction to *The Wounded Healer* by Henri Nouwen (New York: Doubleday, 1979).

3. Bureau of the Census, *65+ in the United States* (Washington, DC: U.S. Department of Commerce, Economic and Statistics Administration, Bureau of the Census, 1996).

4. Family Caregiving in the U.S. (Bethesda, MD: The National Alliance for Caregiving and The American Association of Retired Persons, 1998). Available at: <http://www.caregiving.org/content/reports/finalreport.pdf>. Accessed October 19, 2001.

5. National Alliance for Caregiving. The Caregiving Boom: Baby Boomer Women Giving Care. (Bethesda, MD: National Alliance for Caregiving, 1998). Available at: <http://www.caregiving.org/content/reports/babyboomer.pdf>. Accessed October 15, 2001.

6. Stephen A. Moss, "LTC Choice: A Simple, Cost Free Solution to the Long-Term Care Puzzle," *Public Policy and Aging* (Washington, DC: The Association for Gerontology in Higher Education, 2001), pp. 117-123.

7. Ibid.

8. John Dunlop, "Successful Aging: Living the End of Life to the Glory of God," *Dignity,* 2001, 7(4): 3.

9. Mary Pipher, *Another Country; Navigating the Emotional Terrain of Our Elders* (New York: The Berkely Publishing Group, 1999), p. 77.

10. John F. Kilner, *Life on the Line: Ethics, Aging, Ending Patient's Lives, and Allocating Vital Resources* (Bannockburn, IL: The Center for Bioethics and Human Dignity, 1992), pp. 153-175.

11. George E. Vaillant, *Aging Well: Surprising Guideposts to a Happier Life from the Landmark Harvard Study of Adult Development* (New York, NY: Little, Brown and Company, 2002).

12. Sybil D. Smith, "Theoretical Models of Parish Nursing, Chaplains, and Parish Clergy Interdisciplinary Relationships." In Larry VandeCreek and Sue Mooney (Eds.), *Navigating the Maze of Professional Relationships: Parish Nurses, Health Care Chaplains, and Community Clergy* (Binghamton, NY: The Haworth Press, Inc., 2003), pp. 217-226.

13. Susan H. Taft (2000): "An Inclusive Look at the Domain of Ethics and Its Application to Administrative Behavior," *Online Journal of Issues in Nursing.* Available at: <http://www.nursingworld.org/ojin/topic8/topic8_6.htm>. Accessed December 2, 2002.

14. Ann Solari-Twadell, "The Emerging Practice of Parish Nursing," *Parish Nursing: Promoting Whole Person Health Within Faith Communities* (Thousand Oaks, CA: Sage, 1999), p. 23.

15. Sybil D. Smith, "Six Years of Learning," *The Oates Journal* 3 [online]. Available: <http://www.oates.org/journal/mbr/vol-03-2000/articles/s_smith-sb1.html>.

16. Lynda W. Miller, "Nursing Through the Lens of Faith," *Journal of Christian Nursing,* 1997, 14(1): 17-21.

17. Sybil D. Smith, "Response to God's Life-Giving Ways by Ralph Underwood," *Insights, Austin Seminary Faculty Journal,* 1999, 114(2): 29-32.

18. Sybil D. Smith, "Parish Nursing: A Call to Integrity," *Journal of Christian Nursing,* 2000, 17(1): 18-20.

Chapter 2

Overview of Parish Nursing

Sybil D. Smith

Health ministries is an umbrella term that embraces parish nursing, health promotion, congregational health, and other health-related activities which take place at church sites for congregational members and the community served by the congregation. The Health Ministries Association (HMA) was announced in 1989 as a membership organization. As a membership organization the HMA is a multidisciplinary, interfaith group. The parish nurse section of the HMA in conjunction with the American Nurses Association published the *Scope and Standards of Parish Nursing Practice* in 1998.[1] The purpose of this chapter is to give an overview of parish nursing, clarify terminology, explore the roles for parish nurses within a faith community, and discuss the function of parish nurses in the health system and the effectiveness of parish nurse programs.

SCOPE AND STANDARDS OF PARISH NURSING PRACTICE

A major contribution of the *Scope and Standards of Parish Nursing Practice* is the consensus it brings to some confusing terminology. The following definitions are from that document unless otherwise stated.

Terminology

> *Faith community:* An organization of families and individuals who share common values, beliefs, religious doctrine, and faith practices that influence their lives, such as church, syna-

gogue, or mosque, and that functions as a client system, a focus for parish nursing.

Healing: The process of integrating the body, mind, and spirit to achieve wholeness, health, and a sense of well-being, even when the curing of disease may not occur.

Health: Wholeness, salvation, shalom. The integration of the physical, psychological, social, and spiritual aspects of the client system and harmony with self, others, the environment, and God.

Health Ministry: The promotion of health and healing as part of the mission and ministry of a faith community to its members and the community it serves.

Health Promotion: Activities that persons undertake to achieve desired health outcomes.

Parish Nurse: A registered professional nurse who serves as a member of the ministry staff of a faith community to promote health and wholeness of the faith community and the community it serves.

Health Minister: A health minister is not defined by the document; however, a general consensus is that a health minister is laity or professionals that engage in ministries of health.

Illness: The experience of brokenness; disintegration of body, mind, spirit; and disharmony with others, the environment, and God.

For the purposes of this text the terms *parish nurse* and *congregational nurse* are used interchangeably. The terms *parish* and *church* are also used interchangeably to denote both the membership of a faith community in a collective way and sometimes the physical structures of a faith community. The term *parish nurse program* is used to denote the administrative and operations structure from which parish nurse ministry takes place.

Functions of the Parish Nurse in the Faith Community

Seven functions of the parish nurse are described by Granger Westberg.[2] The functions include health educator, personal health counselor, referral agent, trainer of volunteers, developer of support groups, integrator of faith and health, and health advocate. Through these functions the parish nurse can promote health and wholeness for the local church and the community it serves. These seven functions can play out differently in particular denominations and geographic regions, and are further explicated throughout this book.

A parish nurse program in a church with a strong commitment to parish nursing from the clergy will not look the same as a parish nurse program in a church where the clergy leadership is not familiar with the concept. In Chapter 1, the stories of Koby and Nadine demonstrated the difference. The ease with which Koby implemented a program was not experienced by Nadine. For Nadine, it was like starting over again when the new pastor came on board.

When a parish nurse program unfolds from within a community of faith, the administrative support that can take years to build is already in place. The level of structural support from the denomination headquarters impacts the functions or roles of parish nurses as well as the way effectiveness of a parish nurse program is measured.

Marcia A. Schnorr is the national Coordinator for Parish Nurse Ministry in the Lutheran Church Missouri Synod, which has over 500 parish nurses. In the next section, Marcia relates the development of parish nurse ministry in a denomination in which the idea and support came from the top down.

PARISH NURSE MINISTRY IN THE LUTHERAN CHURCH MISSOURI SYNOD

Marcia A. Schnorr

In the late 1980s Reverend Howard E. Mueller was Executive Director for the Lutheran Church Missouri Synod (LCMS) Health and Healing Group. He and the Committee for Health and Healing took an interest in parish nursing and began planning for its introduction to entities within the LCMS. In winter 1988, I was appointed to the volunteer position of national parish nurse coordinator for LCMS.

When I was first approached to be the national coordinator, my response was, "I didn't know we had a parish nurse ministry." I was told, "We don't, but we'd like to start one." Some of us (nurses) were doing parish nursing before Reverend Mueller recruited for a national coordinator. We were doing so with the blessings of our congrega-

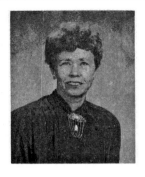

Marcia A. Schnorr, RN, EdD, has been the parish nurse at St. Paul Lutheran Church, Rochelle, Illinois, for over fifteen years. She has been the National Coordinator, Parish Nurse Ministry-Lutheran Church Missouri Synod, for twelve years, serving first in a voluntary capacity and now as paid deployed staff. Schnorr has been a principal mentor for parish nurse students in the parish nurse/distance-learning program from Concordia University in Wisconsin, and an active participant in the Northern Illinois District Lutheran Church Missouri Synod Parish Nurse Network. Dr. Schnorr received her parish nursing and lay ministry education at Concordia University, Wisconsin. She is a frequent speaker at parish nurse conferences. In addition, she teaches community mental health nursing at Kishwaukee College, Malta, Illinois, and provides her nursing students with a brief overview of parish nursing.

tion—sometimes calling it something else besides parish nursing. In the Lutheran Church Missouri Synod the local congregations can have particular areas of ministry without there being something similar on the national level . . . as long as it does not contradict the basic teachings of the denomination.

The formal beginning of the LCMS parish nursing movement began with the announcement of my position and the development of a manual for parish nurses. We produced promotional brochures and promoted parish nursing through exhibits, breakfasts, and break-out sessions at major denominational meetings.

In the early 1990s we experienced some changes in the International Center of the LCMS when the director retired. The new director, Dr. Bruce Hartung, continued to support parish nursing, and parish nursing continued to flourish on both the congregational level and the national level. Our parish nurses began grassroots networking within many of the thirty-five districts that comprise LCMS. The parish nurses had exhibits at the district conventions and pastors' conferences.

At the national level our publications were reviewed, revised, and made available to individuals and groups. A quarterly newsletter was initiated; a national directory of persons involved in congregational health ministry and parish nursing was developed; parish nursing was added to the LCMS Health Ministries Web site <http://humancare. lcms.org/HM/menu.htm>. From this Web site many resources can be accessed, such as a fifty-page manual for parish nursing and the LCMS Standards of Practice for the Parish Nurse. We have encouraged all thirty-five districts to appoint a congregational health ministry/parish nurse district representative. As the national coordinator I serve as a consultant to pastors, nurses, and others interested in parish nursing. I am available for internal consultation, especially with the Lutheran Church in Australia.

Basic, advanced, and continuing education offerings are available through various schools within the LCMS Concordia System and district networks. There is an additional opportunity for parish nurses to enroll in either a lay ministry or deaconess program and become rostered as a professional church worker.

As we move into the new millennium, we continue to experience growth and change. Now I am paid as a part-time deployed staff. Two of us are paid at the national level. The manager of health promotions is a part-time position (two days per week) that includes health pro-

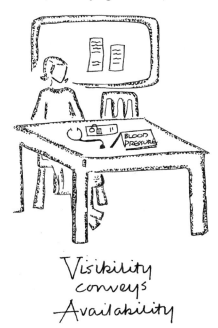

Visibility
conveys
Availability

motions to staff and responsibilities to congregational health ministries/parish nursing. My contract is eight hours per week. So although there are two of us, it is still not a full-time equivalent. Our interest in the whole person and the desire to share the love of Christ through word and deed provides an opportunity for parish nursing to become an accepted part of the ministry within the church both nationally and in individual congregations.

Reflections on Marcia's Story

The denominational structure for parish nursing in the LCMS allowed for the orderly unfolding of a large ministry of health over a fourteen-year period. The underlying philosophy, guiding the process of parish nurse program development, was congruent with the vision of the mission and ministry of the faith tradition itself. The leadership for the program came from within the community of faith and not from outside market values. No doubt parish nurses within the LCMS system turn to local health care organizations for education and resource support; they do not have to seek external sources for instruction on how to do ministry. The necessary support is within

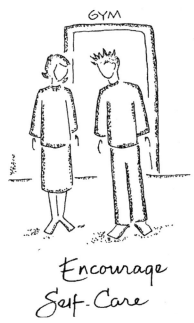

GYM

Encourage
Self-Care

the larger community of faith. The functions of the parish nurse in a congregation-driven program will be the functions the church believes to be important to their purpose and vision.

Functions of the Parish Nurse in the Hospital System

Many parish nurse programs were started in the 1990s when hospitals sought out congregations for partnerships. Some hospitals sponsored paid nurses for congregations and others paid only a hospital parish nurse coordinator to stimulate volunteerism of nurses for their respective congregations. Hospital programs for parish nursing developed often as community outreach during the days of extreme competition in health care. Hospitals started providing services in the community similar to those people expected from the local health departments, and many were provided on site at the church.

Although public health nursing and community health nursing appear on the surface to have focuses similar to parish nursing and health ministry, they are limited in the practice of integrating the spiritual realm of care.[3] Public health nursing is a population-focused practice while community health nurses provide liaisons with com-

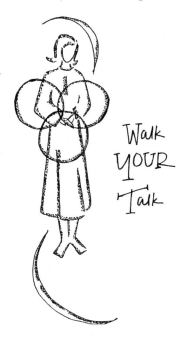

Walk
YOUR
Talk

munity services, make home visits, and incorporate family members into the care of a client.

The function of the parish nurse in a hospital-driven program will be either that of a coordinator of other nurses providing programs in churches, or that of a paid nurse serving a congregation who reports to a hospital-based parish nurse coordinator. Hospitals are entities that want to make decisions based on good science and quantitative research data about the outcomes of programs they finance. Program evaluation and effectiveness measures will not be the same for hospital-based programs as they would be in congregation-based programs. For example, in Marcia's story, the goals and objectives would be very different and expectations for quantitative analysis would be slim.

EFFECTIVENESS OF PARISH NURSE PROGRAMS

The effectiveness of parish nurse programs is addressed in the *Scope and Standards of Parish Nursing Practice* in the Quality of Care Standard of Performance. The standard relates that parish nurses systematically participate in evaluation of the quality and effectiveness of their parish nurse practice. The rationale recognizes that parish nursing is an evolving specialty. Six methods are listed with which to evaluate the effectiveness of parish nurse practice as part of a health ministry in a faith community. The first four methods concern the care rendered and the client population. The last two methods suggested are both about the administrative environment and managerial operations for the parish nurse program: (1) determining the effectiveness in the use of time, energy, and resources to achieve outcomes; and (2) developing policies and procedures to improve the parish nursing practice.[4]

Effectiveness has to do with the ability to produce a desired result. So how do we know when a parish nurse program is effective or has reached a desired result? The answer lies in understanding how decisions are made for the congregation. Consider a systems lens to view the parish nurse program as a smaller organization within the larger organization of congregational ministries, within the larger organization of a congregation itself, which may or may not be part of a larger collective organization of shared values such as a conference, diocese, presbytery, convention, network, etc. Decisions made at the collective level may or may not be binding on the local congregation.

When collective-level decisions are binding on the local congregation, the congregation is thought of as dependent on a hierarchal system. When collective-level decisions are not binding on the local congregation, the congregation is considered to be autonomous and independent in decision making. However, reality teaches that dependent versus independent terms are but the poles on a continuum of decision-making rationale within communities of faith.

Effectiveness of a parish nurse program is tied to the chain for decision making about the program. Stephen Robbins, an organization theorist, has defined organizational effectiveness as the degree to which an organization attains its short- and long-term goals, the selection of which reflects strategic constituencies, the self-interest of the evaluator, and the life stage of the organization.[5] In thinking about the desired results of a parish nurse program being tied to the short- and long-range goals, the question asked is just what goals have to be met to determine effectiveness. Every layer in the internal decision-making chain represents a different group of constituents with goals for the parish nurse program. Another group of constituents or contingencies that need to be satisfied are those external to the community of faith. Outside the community of faith, the professional standards, relevant statutes, and regulations have to be met.[6] More ambiguous are the expectations of health systems and community agencies for parish nurse programs. Sometimes the agendas of health systems and community agencies collide with the values of the congregation. Thinking in terms of multiple contingencies to be satisfied and colliding value systems, the question becomes, Which contingency whose goals are left unmet can threaten the survival of the parish nurse program?

The contingency that could quickly impact survival of the program is the contingency that is more financially committed to the program. For instance, who pays the nurses' salaries? Is it the congregation, the health system, or a community coalition? Only a serious error in judgment would cause a parish nurse program not to make considerable effort to meet the goals of the financial investors of the program. The contingency that is the payment source for the nurse's salary will determine the effectiveness of goals for the use of time, energy, and resources to achieve outcomes.

Policies and procedures must be put in place to complement the goals of the dominant contingency. When the nurse is paid by the congregation or the ecclesiastical body, harmony is less challenged in the faith community. When the nurse is paid by an agency outside the congregation, the parish nurse undertakes a great balancing act to keep multiple contingencies satisfied. Movement toward the goals of the paying contingency are expected, while at the same time the goals of the church leadership are imperative. When the structure for the parish nurse program does not provide the processes necessary to satisfy multiple contingencies, the parish nurse program's ability to influence the lives of the client population is weak. In the past decade parish nursing was evolving in sort of an entrepreneurial way with little structure. The high levels of commitment and creativity displayed by the pioneer parish nurses of the 1990s have endowed parish nursing in the new millennium with a developing organizational structure that will stabilize and sustain parish nurse programs over time.

The following chapter is a story of high commitment and passionate creativity. The writer was completing her doctoral dissertation at the same time the story was unfolding. It was because of her level of readiness, knowledge of systems, and ability to accept uncertainty that she was able to accomplish so much. The historical events taking place in the politics of health care delivery in the 1990s decided the outcomes and rendered a verdict on the integrity and ethics of health system administration in the United States. Spiritual care products entered the marketplace and parish nurse programs became window dressing in more than one health system. Dollar amounts were placed on the number of parish nurse services rendered and the number of participants and tax write-offs that were available in some states on the work of mandated volunteerism. Attempts to genuinely measure outcomes and evaluate effectiveness were near futile in many health system programs.

NOTES

1. Health Ministries Association, Inc. and American Nurses Association, *Scope and Standards of Practice for Parish Nursing* (Washington, DC: American Nurses Publishing, 1998).

2. Granger Westberg, "A Personal Historical Perspective of Whole Person Health and the Congregation," In Phyllis Ann Solari-Twadell and Mary Ann McDermott (Eds.), *Parish Nursing: Promoting Whole Person Health in Faith Communities.* (Thousand Oaks, CA: Sage, 1999), pp. 35-41.

3. Peggy S. Matteson, "A New Yet Old Model of Care," *Massachusetts Nurse,* 1999, 69(3): 5.

4. Health Ministries Association, *Scope and Standards,* p. 16.

5. Stephen P. Robbins, *Organizational Theory: Structure, Design, and Application* (Englewood Cliffs, NJ: Prentice-Hall, 1990), p. 77.

6. Health Ministries Association, *Scope and Standards,* p. 16.

Chapter 3

A Spirit of Commitment and Creativity

Renae Schumann

Outcome effectiveness is measured by standards developed or understood by the interested parties. When multiple entities such as a hospital system, nursing schools, community agencies, and numerous faith communities (churches) are involved in development of volunteer programs and projects, measurement of outcome effectiveness can be difficult. Of greatest concern is deciding which objectives should be considered the standard for effectiveness. When entity objectives are not congruent, measurement becomes meaningless and cumbersome, and the program seems ineffective.

The following tells the story of one hospital-based volunteer congregational health program and the consideration of effectiveness. The mission of the hospital system at the onset of the program, and therefore of the congregational nurse program, included providing

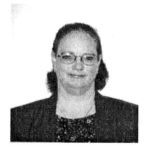
Renae Schumann, PhD, RN, is Assistant Professor for clinical nursing at the University of Texas Health Science Center at Houston School of Nursing where she teaches baccalaureate and graduate students. She is also the volunteer congregational nurse for her home church. Previously she was Director of Congregational Outreach for Memorial Hermann Healthcare System in Houston. She received her bachelor of science in nursing and her master of science in nursing from the University of Texas Health Science Center at Houston and her doctor of philosophy degree from Texas Woman's University—Houston Center.

health education and care to underserved populations. All hospital system employee performance appraisals included a requirement of volunteer community service at the outset of the congregational health program. However, time and economic challenges refocused the hospital system from benevolent programs to income-generating programs and projects. The focus of the congregational nursing program shifted from offering a ministry of health and improving access to health services, to a pure marketplace model.

THE BEGINNINGS

Parish nursing was a hot commodity in the 1990s. Hospitals and churches each wanted their own parish nurse program so they could match the program of the group down the street. Our hospital system was no different. The director of the pastoral care department heard about parish nursing through local pastors and hospital administrators. He was determined to establish a program for his multifacility, faith-based hospital system. He contacted me at the neighboring faith-based school of nursing because I was involved in developing curriculum for a graduate program in parish nursing. We established a committee for the purpose of writing a proposal for a hospital-based congregational nurse program, which would serve the area immediately surrounding the school.

The First Proposal

Our committee included the director of pastoral care for the six satellite hospitals of the health system, the director of nursing from the largest of the hospitals, and myself from the nursing school. The proposal was written as a pilot project to include a partnership arrangement with three major groups, namely the hospital, the nursing school, and the participating churches. If the pilot year of the program was considered successful, then the project would expand to include the other five satellite hospitals and the churches supported by those hospitals.

The proposal detailed job descriptions for a full-time paid parish nurse coordinator who would work in the pastoral care department of the source hospital. A volunteer committee chairperson from each participating satellite hospital would serve as an advisor to the coordinator. The purpose of the proposed project was to provide health education and a few health promotion projects to identified "at-risk" area churches. Program resources were to come from the hospital and the nursing school. Programs and services would be free of charge to the churches. Occasional support would be enlisted from community agencies.

The proposal was presented to administrators of the hospital system, the nursing school, and the university of which the nursing school was a part. Unfortunately, the congregational and parish nursing concept was still unclear to the hospital administrators in the meeting. The hospital system rejected the proposal on the grounds that it seemed too risky to support, even in the pilot stage. The university, and therefore the nursing school, rejected the proposal. Although the hospital system and the university shared the same faith base and both received funding from the same denominational body, the university administration was hesitant to commit faculty and students to a project they were not confident the Board of Regents would support.

A few weeks later I received a call from the health system pastoral care director. He related that he had simplified the proposal and pre-

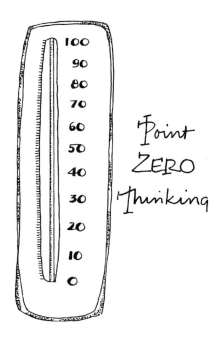

sented it again to the health system administrators, and they were willing to try the project for a period of three years if sufficient funding and a coordinator who had knowledge of parish nursing, education, systems operations, and team leadership could be located.

I accepted the job as coordinator and filled the spot as a full-time employee of the health system in the pastoral care department. Since administration had guaranteed a three-year program, I was able to focus on the six-satellite hospital system instead of targeting the area surrounding the source hospital where I was located. I began to think about a more comprehensive program that would deliver services to the entire city instead of one portion of the city. On my first day I was promoted from hospital program coordinator to system program director. The move gave me the administrative authority to recruit and lead multidisciplinary teams systemwide instead of being limited to nursing teams in one hospital. The following describes the newly created Congregational Outreach Program.

THE CONGREGATIONAL OUTREACH PROGRAM

The Congregational Outreach Program or COP, as it was called, was part of the systemwide Pastoral Care Department, so I, as director, was considered a system employee, not a satellite hospital employee. This status gave me access to all of the hospitals and resources they had to offer. The organizational structure developed for the COP reflected system participation (see Figure 3.1).

Organizational Structure

Hospital Volunteers

The COP was staffed strictly by hospital employee volunteers. Approximately 80 percent of the volunteers for church events such as health fairs or screening programs were registered nurses, physical therapists, lab technicians, or chaplains. Most of the volunteers for church events came from within the congregation being served, if possible, or from the satellite hospital which served that area. For example, if the church event was located in the southwest part of the city, hospital volunteers came from the southwest area hospital to staff that event.

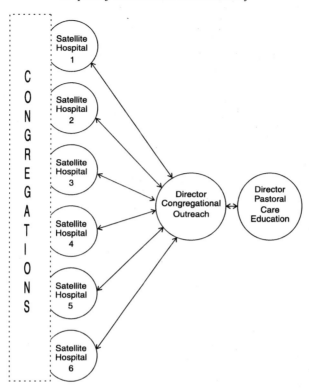

FIGURE 3.1. Congregational Outreach Program

For the first three years of the program, volunteers from hospital staff were easy to find. Employee annual performance appraisals held a community service component, which meant that 5 percent of the evaluation was based on the amount of community service the employee had performed within the past year. When hospital or system employees volunteered at COP events they received a thank-you letter for their employee file. My signature as director made the form official and the employee was given credit for community service. Community service credit ultimately contributed to greater salary increases for participating employee volunteers so recruiting volunteer staff for church functions was not a problem. I often had a waiting list of employees who were eager to complete community service requirements before their annual review.

The Steering Committee

The COP was a health system program based in the health system pastoral care department. This relationship provided one automatic link within each satellite hospital, namely the hospital chaplain. Through the chaplains I was able to meet key people in each facility and to establish a network of supporters. These supporters became a steering committee that advised me in volunteer recruitment and utilization of system resources. Each committee member had been with the system for several years and was familiar with the politics, easiest route to success, and the keepers of the red tape. The steering committee met quarterly so that programs could be planned and developed.

The Subcommittee

Each steering committee member served as the chair to a subcommittee specific to the needs of his or her respective hospital and area of town. Subcommittees were comprised of interested employees, area pastors, and community leaders. The purpose of the subcommittees was to keep me informed of parish nursing activities and the needs of their churches. I met with each subcommittee quarterly, then generated a report to deliver to the steering committee.

After the subcommittees had been structured, participating congregations were recruited. We found the churches by surveying the system employees regarding their interest in providing health programs to their own faith communities. Seventy employees completed the survey and facilitated meetings with their church leaders. Hospital employee involvement in the meetings indicated commitment to the COP and every effort was made to fulfill their request for those programs quickly.

Pastors and Churches

Initial meetings with pastors or church leaders proved fruitful. Churches were mapped geographically and the satellite hospital closest to the church provided the human and material resources for the event. Examples of beginning programs included health fairs, and classes on CPR, living wills, power of attorney, and healthy cooking. For each specialized program such as the living wills or cooking classes, experts from within the congregations were recruited to teach. One church had a probate attorney among its membership who agreed to teach a two-hour class on the will package. Church leaders opened the class to the community so that it could be used as an outreach program as well. Several nonmembers attended the class and eventually began attending the church services.

Case Study

A registered nurse employee from the southwest area hospital indicated on the survey that she would be interested in establishing a parish nursing program in her middle-class church. She and I met with the pastor and we decided to perform an assessment of the church members' perceived health needs within two weeks. It was agreed that the nurse would distribute the survey forms during the Sunday Bible class period and collect the completed forms for at least a week. Afterward, I would compile the results of the survey. Then she, the pastor, and I would discuss the results to determine the type of programming that would best suit the needs of the congregation.

Although we had intended to focus primarily on the adults, the youth group class (ages twelve to eighteen) also completed the forms. This age group listed stress management, grief, and bereavement as their perceived priority health education needs.

I spoke with the nurse about these findings, but she knew nothing about the youth group or its dynamics. We scheduled another appointment with the pastor and the youth minister, during which time we learned that the youth group had experienced three suicides within the past year. The youth minister was surprised that the youth recognized those needs and were emotionally comfortable enough to acknowledge those feelings in writing. The four of us began planning appropriate programming for the group and the remainder of the congregation, and the pastor asked the nurse if she would consider going through educational processes to become the parish nurse so that similar projects could be developed as needed.

We developed an event specific to the identified need of the church. After discussing the options with the pastor, the youth minister, and the new parish nurse, it was decided to have open sessions with social workers. One of the system's adolescent population social workers spoke to the youth during the Sunday evening youth group meeting, and an adult care social worker spoke with the parents separately during the same time period. Both groups were given information regarding teen suicide, including assessment of risk factors and potential interventions.

Program evaluation indicated that both groups appreciated the information given but, more important, that they were grateful that someone had taken the time to develop the event for them. The teens stated that they had wanted to talk to someone about their grief, fear, and stress so they were appreciative about the social worker's class. Many of them sought additional help, and many parents learned to better recognize signs of teen depression or suicidal ideation. The church considered the program a success and began to assess for further program needs and opportunities. The nurse attended continuing education classes on parish nursing concepts to become more efficient at applying nursing process to the congregation setting.

Outcome effectiveness was easily measured. The church's objective was to provide information and resources which promoted the spiritual and emotional health of its members. The COP and hospital system objectives were to serve the community by delivering quality health and wellness education to faith communities free of charge. The program was deemed effective and successful.

CREATIVE GROWTH

The COP began to grow very quickly and human and material resources were in great demand. There were always multiple projects in all parts of town. The steering committee and subcommittees met often, and each meeting flowed with rich dialogue and creative brainstorming in an effort to efficiently serve the greatest number of people within the city of four million. It became obvious that the COP structure was not strong enough to support the rapid growth, even with active committee participation. I was still the only paid person in COP, and all other human resources were hospital employee volunteers.

Keeping up with COP growth and popularity was challenging. After making the initial contacts with the pastors of hospital employees who had completed the surveys, COP had enough to keep constantly busy. There was an apparent "health fair epidemic" during which time each church wanted its own health fair or similar event.

The more programs the COP developed, the greater the need became for its services. Events and opportunities were continuous, and they became more refined and focused to the perceived needs as I became better at assessment and planning. For example, one church had many expectant mothers at the same time. Many of the moms had little or no experience regarding infants or child care so I developed a special event, a baby fair, to address parent education. Exhibitors included hospital nursery nurses, labor and delivery nurses, lactation consultants, nutritionists, safety experts to teach proper installation of car seats, toy experts, etc. We even had a scrapbook consultant. Parents learned to bathe and dress babies, to properly feed them, to administer medications, and much more. The parents enjoyed the program and stated that the only problem was that it was too short.

Two years later we planned a safety fair for those same growing families. During this event parents and kids learned about stranger danger, water safety, fire hazards, bicycle safety, and more. Again, families enjoyed the event and were grateful for what they had learned.

Effectiveness of these events was measured by the hospital system and by the church. Hospital system objectives were met because most of the volunteers of both programs were recruited from the hospitals while the remainder came from the community. Material resources were free of charge to the church and the community. Church objectives were met because the leaders and the parish nurse wanted to provide low-cost programming to benefit the needs of young families. Both events were well publicized and open to the community, and nonmembers attended. New families started to attend worship services regularly, which contributed to church growth. These programs were considered effective and successful.

CREATIVE RESOURCES

Eventually the hospital system resources, both human and material, started to burn out and events were more difficult to manage. Event scheduling did not cease, and new churches entered the program every week. The health and wellness education needs of the

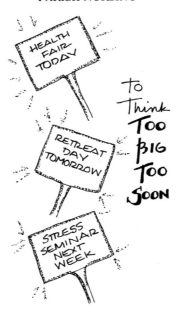

large city loomed over the COP. There was so much work to do, so little time, and so few resources.

Resources from the Churches

Event volunteers had to start coming more often from within the congregation or from community agencies. COP focus turned more heavily toward recruiting church volunteers to staff multidisciplinary health ministry programs. The parish nurses who had participated in small parish nursing education programs were encouraged to identify resources within the church first, then the community, then the health care system. Parish nurse education programs gave detailed descriptions on how to find and keep volunteers.

Large churches could easily staff their own events. Smaller churches, however, had a more difficult time. I was still the only paid parish nurse in a program of nearly 100 active churches, so I required that all churches staff the nontechnical aspects of events while I staffed or outsourced the more technical aspects.

The policy was revised with time, and soon churches holding one event were encouraged to provide volunteers for an event held at another church. Common practice became a volunteer chain in which volunteers from one church helped with the next event that was held at another church. Eventually volunteers were crossing ethnic, economical, geographic, and denominational boundaries to help others. Their willingness to help the other churches gave them access to the resources that were becoming more scarce. Knowing that their church's needs were being addressed motivated them to serve others in the community.

In some instances suburban middle-class churches that supported in-town mission churches would draw from their members to support the health ministry needs of the mission church. One multithousand-member church supported approximately twenty mission churches within the city. Members of the large church regularly visited the missions and offered various forms of support. A health ministry program was developed in which members of the large, sponsoring church provided health ministry programs to the mission sites. One mission church had several attendees who allowed their children to skip school and play on the streets. When asked why this was happening, the mission director explained the parents were primarily immigrants who did not understand the school system. They would not get the children immunized and, as a result, the children could not go to school. People from the sponsoring large church developed a mentoring program in which they helped more functional parents of the mission church teach the less functional parents. In this way, parents developed an understanding of and appreciation for immunizations and school attendance.

In contrast to this mission model was another smaller mission church supported by approximately twenty-five area churches. Members of the sponsoring churches often reported to the mission church to help with the homeless population, the food pantry, the clothes closet, etc. Members of the support churches easily adapted to providing health and wellness needs for the mission church.

One summer the children of the mission church needed health screenings and immunizations for the school year. There were no resources to pay for this service and church leaders were concerned about the possibility of getting the children into the church for such an event. We established the Youth Group Bazaars to draw the children and their families to the event. Youth groups from the supporting churches came to the mission church and set up carnival-like booths for games and prizes. The city health department and volunteers from the supporting churches donated time and supplies to provide screening and immunizations to children before they entered the booth area. Many children were immunized that day so that they could go to school, and the various youth groups reported having an "awesome" time with the mission church's kids.

Resources from Education Provided for Parish Nurses

Another valuable source of volunteers was provided by the continuing education programs that I held five to six times per year for those wanting to learn about parish nursing. Each program had several participants so I made announcements regarding the current needs and asked for help. It was a rare occasion that my requests were unfilled during these "caring calls." My favorite example occurred during one summer program when I was able to recruit volunteer nursing staff for three church health fairs, and find a volunteer to accompany bike riders on a 400-mile trip to raise money for their medical missions.

Many of the same parish nurses attended the education programs and they were accustomed to asking one another for help and to using their church and agency resources to serve other parish nurses and the greater community. They would often come with their own caring call lists to share with one another. We each did what we could to help others provide resources for church events.

Resources from the Community

The COP became known for designing and presenting customized programming, and I received numerous calls weekly from church leaders who were interested in participating in health ministry activities. I became adept at planning, developing, and leading multidisciplinary teams to implement large multifacility and multiagency projects. The best example is Diabetes Sunday, during which the hospital system and volunteers, the American Diabetes Association, a medical equipment manufacturer, and a local newspaper partnered to provide blood glucose screening for thirteen area African-American churches. At the end of the four-hour multisite event, fifteen hospital volunteers, thirty church volunteers, and five community agency volunteers had provided blood glucose screening, education, and referrals to nearly 400 people.

Effectiveness of the Diabetes Sunday was difficult to determine. There were so many different entities involved and so many different agendas. There were many more people to screen than there were people to do the screening, so some potentially at-risk churchgoers left without being screened. Despite my best efforts to recruit hospital volunteers, only a handful agreed to give up part of their Sunday to help. Most of the hospital employee volunteers were diabetic educators or members of one of the test-site churches. The novelty of the COP was wearing off and hospital employees were anxious to spend their time elsewhere.

The hospital system's focus was shifting from providing free access to its resources to being reimbursed for any service performed. Although the 400 screened individuals were referred to the hospital system if necessary, administrators saw little benefit in any program which did not produce immediate tangible results. According to the hospital system, the Diabetes Sunday project was ineffective.

The leaders and members of the test-site churches were disappointed that so few volunteers had come to help their congregations. Some of the pastors stated that limitations in the number of health care workers had proven only to frustrate their members, thus making the church administrators "look bad" for agreeing to host the event. The majority of the church leaders considered the Diabetes Sunday project ineffective because it seemed to be more trouble than it was worth.

Four hundred people were screened in a four-hour period. Of the 400 screened, 130 were identified as potential Type 2 diabetics. Therefore, the Diabetes Association and those identified considered the project very effective. The medical supply company which donated the necessary equipment and the local newspaper which publicized the event considered the project effective because their respective names had been brought before the community.

Diabetes Sunday was an extraordinary amount of work, especially in the fourth year of COP operation. The difficulty in recruiting volunteers, the number of meetings with pastors and church volunteers, the meetings with the other community agencies, the grant writing for the equipment donation, transport of signage and equipment to the sites prior to the event, and site visits during the event proved challenging yet educational.

Important to know is that the other COP activities did not stop during Diabetes Sunday; rather, several other events ran simultaneously. In addition to the large event were two health fairs and three special class sessions which I had arranged through the hospital system's Speaker's Bureau. Since I was still the only paid employee in the COP, and because of the extreme work which had to be done to ensure success, I believed that despite the 130 identified, the Diabetes Sunday event was not as effective as it could have been had more people been available to help with the preparations, the actual event, or the other COP activities.

WHAT WENT WRONG

The Congregational Outreach Program was a good idea. Many health and wellness education needs were met citywide, and hundreds of people received services in the form of various health screenings and referrals, specialized education programs, flu shots, and health ministry program implementation. The COP started with nothing—no resources, no churches, no volunteers or staff—and by the end of the nearly four operational years had developed or assisted in developing health ministry programs in 150 churches citywide. Even six years after its beginning, fifty of those health ministry programs are still functioning.

In addition to the health ministry program development, educational programs providing the basics of parish nursing and health ministry implementation were taught a total of twenty-five times across the state during the four years of service. Additional offerings with greater focus on mental health care in the church, legal and ethical issues, and spiritual assessment and care were presented periodically.

As good as the COP had been, it could not survive the economic and financial changes that the hospital system experienced. Despite efforts to continue the program, COP was neither strong enough nor well enough supported within the system to maintain operation. There were numerous problems with COP structure, funding, staffing, and service provision.

Structure

Any program with scope as broad as the COP must have adequate structure to support that scope. The original structure of the steering committee and the subcommittees became cumbersome with the rapid growth. Efforts to use these committees as program staff were unrealistic because committee members had full-time work responsibilities and COP budget provided only one salary.

Passing time, extraordinary program growth, and difficulty securing resources rendered the committee structure ineffective and obsolete. During years three and four of COP operation, the committees attempted to regroup as one large committee with some participation from each satellite hospital, but those efforts failed. Besides the growth, a major disruption to the committees was the sale of one hospital and acquisition of others. Not only did these changes affect the COP structure, they contributed to internal environment changes which could not be overcome.

Funding

Funding for COP including salary, educational program costs, supplies, and travel came from a grant issued by the hospital system's community services tithe. Each year I reapplied for this grant and was funded for a total of four years. At the end of year three, however, financial difficulties within the system caused the elimination of the community services tithe and closure of all programs the community tithe supported.

When word came that the community tithe was going to end, I attempted to secure funding from other sources. No particular entity could provide funding to support the COP in the way it had been operating. Private funding requirements included focus on one specific part of town or one population instead of accessibility throughout the city and across ethnic and denominational boundaries.

In addition, some of the potential funding agencies stated that although they were impressed by a nurse with advanced degrees directing a large project like COP, they preferred a coordinator who displayed less creativity to focus on a small project within set guidelines. Some said specifically that they saw no need for the "overeducated" staff who could so easily do their jobs. In other words, I was considered a threat by some of the potential funding agencies.

Staffing

While the health system community service requirement mandated employee volunteerism, staffing events had not been difficult. However, the mandated requirement for volunteerism was lifted just as the COP experienced its greatest rate of growth. Lack of volunteers made holding church events impossible at times, which is the reason for creating the caring calls and the volunteer chains. Without those methods the COP would have dissolved much sooner than it did.

Service Provision

In the beginning, services flowed freely because it was part of the hospital system's mission to provide services to the community free of charge. In fact, administrators asked me to find a few underserved churches and suggested we focus on providing as many services as possible. There was a stated interest in my convincing pastors or other church leaders to persuade congregants to seek health care only at system facilities despite individual insurance or employee benefit packages.

As the financial downturn became more problematic and money became scarce, so were the services. I was forced to use community agency resources instead of hospital system resources. This, too, was expensive for the churches and for the COP because often the appropriate agency for the perceived need also invoiced its services. It was just as difficult to resource the community agency service. At times church members agreed to pay nominal fees for service, but those occasions were few and far between and occurred only within middle-income level or higher congregations. Eventually, administrators asked me to charge churches for COP services in order for them to remain active members of the program.

The turning point of COP effectiveness occurred when the economic and financial troubles forced the health system to remove the community service volunteer requirement for employees and limit material resources. These led to decline not only of volunteers to staff events but to elimination of programs to offer the community. As I look back, the organizational structure was too weak to support even a healthily financed project. Even if COP had been better funded, it still needed stronger administrative support and recognition to be truly successful.

CONCLUSION AND FUTURE CREATIVITY

The main lesson learned from the COP experience is easy. Parish nurses or health ministers in any setting, whether congregational or institutional, must be paid. I was the only paid parish nurse in a large, multi-facility, 150-church program based in a not-for-profit hospital system, and the lack of paid staff was detrimental to the program.

Obvious is the connection between funding and securing staff for church events. Volunteers in parish nursing and health ministry projects have a definite place but should not be considered the sole compliment. There were many times when I feared event failure because I could not be sure whether the volunteers would change their minds about staffing an event. Likewise, reimbursed services are more likely to be performed or rendered than are services provided free of charge. When the service well runs dry, those populations in need do without.

Parish nursing programs of the future, whether based in hospitals or churches, will out of necessity be paid positions. Parish nurses are attuned to the aging congregations and the needs of the senior population. Programming for the future must include content such as end-of-life care, lifestyle changes in elder age, and dealing with the stress and fear that often accompany old age. Blood pressure fluctuations causing administration of, or change in, medications are cause for concern, as are adaptations to changes in elimination and other bodily habits. The delivery of service at the individual level will possibly become more important than population-focused program events.

Chapter 4

From the Westberg Project
to the New Millennium

Sybil D. Smith

This chapter presents a summary of the Westberg project and its outgrowth, the International Parish Nurse Resource Center. The role of the Health Ministries Association is discussed and educational pathways for parish nursing are presented with nursing education issues in general as the backdrop.

HISTORY

Parish nursing in the United States emerged from a vision of Granger Westberg, a chaplain and professor at the University of Chicago Medical School.[1] In the late 1970s and early 1980s, Westberg was involved in a project funded by the W. K. Kellogg Foundation, which experimented with physicians' offices operating from church sites. Westberg noticed that nurses were the glue that seemed to hold the communications together between the physicians, the clergy, and the patient. As the W. K. Kellogg project was drawing to a close, Westberg went to the Lutheran General Hospital in Park Ridge, Illinois, where he designed the first hospital-based parish nurse project in 1984. Six Chicago-area churches in conjunction with Lutheran General Hospital hired nurses the following year. Westberg is legitimately acknowledged as the spark behind today's parish nursing; however, meeting the holistic needs of the community of believers has been a part of the Christian church since its inception.[2]

It was Westberg's desire to stimulate dialogue between science and religion at the grassroots level. Westberg envisioned churches as a natural setting, and "spiritually mature" parish nurses as natural organizers for promoting the integration and well-being of mind, body, and spirit.[3] As integrators of faith and health, parish nurses were encouraged to take on functional roles as health educators, personal health counselors, facilitators and resource persons, and trainers of volunteers. The Lutheran General project drew much interest and a year later the National Parish Nurse Resource Center was developed by the Lutheran General Health System. In 1996 it became the International Parish Nurse Resource Center (IPNRC). The Lutheran General Health System is now known as Advocate Health Care. In October 2001, the International Parish Nurse Resource Center was transferred by Advocate Health Care to the Deaconess Foundation of St. Louis, Missouri.

Under new ownership the IPNRC continues to bring nurses together once a year for the Westberg Symposium and promotes continuing education offerings for parish nursing. The Health Ministries Association (HMA) was announced in 1989 as a membership organization with a commitment to promoting parish nursing as a specialized practice of the discipline of nursing and health ministries. As a membership organization the HMA is a multidisciplinary, interfaith group. The American Nurses Association recognized the HMA and jointly published the *Scope and Standards of Parish Nursing Practice* in 1998.[4] The document defines a parish nurse as a registered professional nurse who serves as a member of the ministry staff of a faith community to promote health and wholeness of the faith community and the community it serves.[5]

In the late 1990s the IPNRC plunged into the development of a core curriculum for parish nurse education. The core curriculum was marketed as an "endorsed" curriculum as the IPNRC tried to standardize parish nurse education. Pressure for all parish nurse education programs to become endorsed by the IPNRC created tension in the ranks.[6] What was formerly known as the endorsed core curriculum program is now known as a standardized program with the new owners of IPNRC. Most are offered as a five- to eight-day program usually held in a retreat setting. Not all denominations have provided educational opportunities within the denomination for those experiencing "a call" to parish nursing. The complexity of nurse education has to be considered for a parish nurse program to be properly executed, assuming that the congregation is led by God to take on such ministry.

PARISH NURSE EDUCATION

Issues within nursing can impact what a nurse can bring to parish nurse ministry. Nursing has a historical hierarchical structure, and is a publicly regulated discipline. Until very recently, education for nurses was deficit in processes that promote self-awareness and self-understanding. Reflective learning and theological contemplation are not traditional methods for nursing education even though they are essential to effective ministry. How does a nurse with aspirations of becoming a parish nurse learn these things?

Nursing Issues in General

There are disciplinary inequities within nursing that revolve around the level of education the nurse has completed before first entering nursing practice. It is requisite to discuss entry into practice for nurses because it contributes to the identity of the nurse. There are three basic pathways into nursing practice: (1) the two-year associate degree, (2) the three-year diploma, and (3) the four-year baccalaureate degree (BSN). Graduates from all three pathways are eligible to sit for the same licensing exam that, upon passing, generates the credential of Registered Nurse (RN). From all three pathways the graduate can become a registered nurse, but only at the BSN four-year degree is the nurse known as a professional nurse.[7] Although associate and diploma nurses can carry the RN licensing credential, they are considered to be technical nurses.[8] Within the discipline of nursing, the prolonged lack of resolve over the entry into practice dilemma for nurses is considered by some to be morally unacceptable.[9]

The focus of the technical education process is learning the tasks and technical skills of the trade in preparation for bedside jobs in hospitals. Conceptual thinking is implied within the course work of technical education. In the four-year BSN entry into practice, conceptual course work is explicit at a generalist level. The BSN nurse may work at the bedside but is also prepared to work in the home and community.[10] It is at the graduate specialty level of the nursing master's degree preparation that nurses are, in a meaningful context, educated about conceptual ways of viewing the world.

Tensions exist within nursing because the significance of varied pathways to nursing practice lose meaning when there is a nursing shortage. Often when nurses are in short supply minimum qualifications for a job will be waived, and a technically prepared nurse will be placed into a role requiring skills that are available only from a professional or advanced (master's) degree pathway. Maturity in years and spiritual development of the nurse can sometimes balance the discrepancy. Nurses who gravitate to roles for which they are not academically prepared contend with issues of acceptance from within and without nursing, even when the nurse has an outstanding performance record.[11] Spiritual maturity can assist the nurse in finding a comfort zone; however, the comfort zone can become fragile when new stretches are required.

ENTRY INTO PRACTICE

The entry into practice issue within the nursing profession underscores that all nurses are not equal when they enter an interdisciplinary environment such as health ministries or parish nursing. Some nurses will be more comfortable than others. Good relationship skills can only take one so far when specific knowledge is needed. Along with entry into practice issues and quantitative accountability traditions, nurses are socialized to be others-directed, without a voice of their own.[12] While being others-directed, nurses often practice from a position of authority that inadvertently ignores the client's story and disregards the client's wisdom and agency. Only in recent decades have qualitative methods of knowing been valued in nursing. Opportunities contributing to self-awareness and self-understanding are rare in nursing. Educational methods in nursing do not reinforce a student becoming open to his or her own experience of nursing.[13] Student nurses reflect upon whether it "was the right intervention delivered to the right patient at the right time," and not about what the nurse felt or experienced during the interaction. Nurses do not get to affirm their humanity as part of vocation formation, and the need to reframe disappointments, stress, and discouragement in a positive light goes unmet.[14]

Relationship of Nurse Entry into Practice and Parish Nurse Education

Parish nurse education as endorsed by the original owners of the IPNRC would be considered a commodity in the marketplace. The

IPNRC developed nursing continuing education courses for parish nurses and educators of parish nurses, referring to their courses as "the endorsed" curriculum. Many good continuing education courses emerged in the 1990s, but only those that partnered with the IPNRC could be promoted as the "endorsed curriculum." One must examine whose interests are being served by a self-endorsed program. Do the associate two-year degree nurse, the three-year diploma nurse, the four-year bachelor-degree nurse, and the graduate-degree nurse all need the same introductory course to serve as a parish nurse or health minister? Bethune and Wellard caution against the comodification of education that is vocational in nature.[15] Many variables such as program objectives of the sponsoring congregation can impact the educational pathway needed by a parish nurse.

PARISH NURSING AND HEALTH CARE POLITICS

During the same time that parish nursing was emerging in the United States, the health care industry became focused on combating lifestyle illnesses such as cancer, stroke, heart disease, liver disease, and

" What we
learn will come
up again and
again
in ourselves as
long as we live.
We will be
tested and
examined
over the years
to see if we
understood
what we
have learned."

— Robert Fulghum

accidents. Reducing the economic impact of the effects of lifestyle illness launched the wellness promotion movement of the 1980s. The health promotion/wellness movement appealed to those who valued control and individual choice. The assumption is that individual decisions to participate in cognitive and behavioral health promoting lifestyle strategies can give control over one's health status. Ignored by the lifestyle existential illnesses perspective is that economic, social, cultural, and spiritual factors also contribute to health status. In the early 1990s, while many health care dollars focused on individualistic approaches for lifestyle changes, the epidemics of violence, suicide, unemployment, divorce, and loneliness—the existential illnesses— were building. These existential illnesses, with all of their consequences, impact the bottom line in health care to a greater degree than the lifestyle illnesses. The consequences of existential illness can contribute to physical, emotional, and spiritual brokenness for years after an episode. Unresolved grief and emotional baggage can cross generations.[16]

Health promotion and wellness intervention strategies began to shift from the foreground to the background in the mid-1990s because evidence was weak to support changed behaviors or outcomes. Recognition that change in individual habits and behaviors was spiritual in nature and had to be considered in relationship with family and community came to the forefront. Holistic approaches became popular. The parish nurse movement, while it remained faith based, contributed to whole-person health. The parish nurse programs had aesthetic appeal, and non–faith-based institutions began to launch parish nurse programs in the 1990s.[17]

Advocates for the poor and underserved, such as community development practitioners, along with hospital community service departments envisioned church-based health ministries as an opportunity to expand access to health care for those without health insurance. Expectations of the vision was that middle-class churches would invest in providing health services to those without insurance. Numerous partnerships developed between faith and health groups, but outcomes remain very inconclusive. Discrepancy in underlying substance and structure of various types of parish nurse ministries began to emerge and are further described in the next chapter. It is easy to look back now and see the bigger picture of what was taking place in the 1990s, but for the nurs-

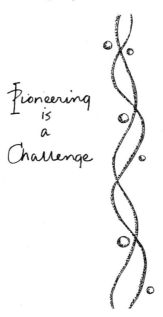

ing pioneers who blazed the trail we build on today, it took grace to go without sight and certainty.

PIONEERING STORIES

The following stories are told by parish nurse coordinators from three different types of parish nurse programs. Bea's and Gerri's stories are about volunteer parish nurse program development. Dana relates a story about developing a hospital-based paid program.

Bea Keller: Parish Nursing in Kentuckiana

The Ohio River may separate the land and the states of Kentucky and Indiana, but it does not separate their parish nurses. Kentuckiana nurses of various religious denominations have heard the call and now minister to their congregations. Concerns about working, ministering, and learning together within or across denominations are unnoticed.

Parish nursing began January 1992 in Louisville, Kentucky, at St. Anthony Hospital with Marge Novi as its first and only parish nurse minister. Her job description required time equally divided be-

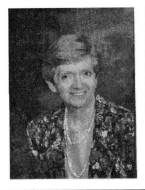

Bea Keller, RN, is a Sister of Charity of Nazareth, Kentucky, and an instructor of the parish nurse certificate program of Spaulding University. Bea is also a doctoral candidate in education at Spaulding. She received a master's in Holistic Health Education from John Kennedy University, Orinda, California, and a BSN from Mercy College of Detroit.

tween an inner city parish, where she would function as parish nurse, and the sponsoring institutions, where she would participate in outreach activities. Marge held the position until 1994, when she resigned and the hospital decided not to replace her immediately. Due to financial problems, the hospital eventually closed in March of 1996.

As with most new programs, it was a learn-as-you-go situation. Marge tried various methods and locations. Initially the base of operations for Marge was in a church office; from there she moved to an office in St. Anthony Hospital and then to an Archdiocese of Louisville office. With each move, some problems were solved while others surfaced.

One of the biggest problems seemed to be explaining the vision of parish nursing to local church and health care personnel. Success stories of parish nurses were plentiful in the Chicago and Milwaukee areas, but the vision was not translating to the Kentuckiana area. Most pastors were already overwhelmed with ideas for various programs, and even if they understood the concept of parish nursing, they did not feel they could take on something new. The other difficulty centered on nurses who were already working and did not have time to give or lacked the understanding of how their nursing skills could be utilized within a church setting.

In September 1993, I began employment at Saints Mary and Elizabeth Hospital located in Louisville. With the title parish nurse coordinator, my job description called for the establishment of a network of volunteer parish nurses who would meet the needs of the newly discharged as well as prospective patients.

My first project was to design a parish nurse program at the neighboring Catholic church. The entire staff of SS. Simon and Jude Catholic Church was very supportive and openly welcomed me to weekly staff meetings. The congregation, on the other hand, had many questions about the need and function of a nurse within their church.

Monthly blood pressure checks before and after church services usually proved a good and understandable way to demonstrate the role of parish nursing to its members. The computer in the church office provided me with a list of twenty-eight nurses who were members of the congregation. These nurses were then invited to a meeting to discuss their role in this new ministry.

Out of the twenty-eight nurses invited, twelve attended; a few others, although unable to attend, expressed their support and desire to be included in future plans. These nurses were excited about using their nursing skills within their church. Many verbalized how as nurses, as well as members of the church, they often felt frustrated in their limitations. They knew the entire nursing process but were limited to making a silent assessment; there was no means allowing them to complete the process. They saw how parish nursing could be the means by which to provide their members with needed health information.

I continued in SS. Simon and Jude Catholic Church for a year. The monthly blood pressure screenings were a huge success. Members began to line up for readings before the nurse even arrived. Members who came were provided with a card listing their blood pressure as well as guidelines ranging from identifying abnormal readings to the need for an emergency room visit. The blood pressure checks provided parishioners the opportunity to ask a nurse health questions. It also provided the nurse with the time she was looking for to do some teaching or to set a follow-up appointment. In addition, weekly weight-loss classes were held during Lent, and a health booth became a part of the parish picnic. The nurses were also invited to provide health education classes to grades three and seven in the parish school.

Not everything was successful. The exercise classes were short-lived as were the monthly health talks. I also learned how difficult it is to set limits when making home visits. The appointment of an interim pastor was an eye-opener. He did not understand my role as a parish nurse, nor did he want to understand it. Although nothing new was begun during his time, I was able to continue with what had been established. The elimination of staff meetings added to the difficulty and caused me to feel very isolated.

After a year at SS. Simon and Jude Catholic Church the concept of parish nursing was introduced to the next church. I began using the same method that had been successful but soon discovered that every church has its own demographics and personality. What worked at SS. Simon and Jude did not work at St. Helen's. Another problem was that the SS. Simon and Jude nurses were very comfortable with me as their coordinator, and none of them felt able to assume the position in my stead.

In 1994, I attended the Parish Nurse Symposium in Park Ridge, Illinois, and in 1996, I completed Phase I and II of a continuing education program and received a certificate in parish nursing from Marquette University in Milwaukee, Wisconsin. The contact with other coordinators and parish nurses was very energizing and provided many new ideas. However, I knew that the Kentuckiana area was different and what was successful elsewhere would not work here. For that reason, I decided not to obtain a faculty certificate from the International Parish Nurse Resource Center.

In September 1996, the Nursing School and the School of Religious Studies at a local Catholic university formed a partnership with the parish nurse program at SS. Mary and Elizabeth Hospital, and the Spalding University Parish Nurse Certificate Program became a reality. The five three-hour sessions were scheduled in the evening for the first Tuesday of the month, from September to May. Topics included "Parish Nursing: What It Is and What It Isn't," "Spirituality of Self-Care, Children, and Youth in the Congregation," "The Older Adult in the Congregation," and "Developing a Parish Nurse Program." Guest speakers provided expert information and gave the concept of parish nursing additional exposure.

Other changes in my position as parish nurse coordinator included providing a one-hour continuing education program on parish nursing for Catholic churches in the area serviced by the hospital, as well as responding to requests of others in the Kentuckiana area. Nurses were then encouraged to begin a program. I would be available as their resource. I am happy to say that many of these programs continue today. The Parish Nurse Support Group began in June 1997 and provided nurses from various churches a monthly opportunity to share their successes and failures. Each meeting also was a forum for problem solving. Six months later, the first issue of the quarterly *Parish Nurse Newsletter* was published, allowing interested nurses to keep up to date with national as well as statewide happenings.

After five years as parish nurse coordinator I resigned. Many changes had taken place within health care. The hospital that hired me had changed its name to Caritas Medical Center and, as with most health care facilities, was having financial problems. I also saw the need to move the program beyond the population stated in my job description. With this in mind, I wrote and received a ministry grant from my religious community, the Sisters of Charity of Nazareth (SCN).

The hospital chose not to replace me, and with the grant I was able to continue in all areas of parish nursing, including the Spalding University Certificate Program, the support groups, and the newsletters. The primary change was the freedom to act as a resource person for Kentuckiana churches of *all* denominations. At this point, I informed SS. Simon and Jude nurses that I would no longer continue coordinating their program. Rather than let it die, three creative nurses decided to divide the various programs among themselves. This alternative continues to work for them.

Since its beginning, the Spalding University Parish Nurse Certificate Program has awarded certificates to over 125 nurses representing Baptist, Episcopal, Lutheran, Presbyterian, Roman Catholic, United Church of Christ, and United Methodist denominations. In January 2000, the university began offering the intermediate parish nurse certificate program. With a two-year format over eight weekends, this program offers parish nurses the opportunity, with directors of religious education, candidates for the deaconate, youth ministers, and other church staff, to learn more about the theological foundations of ministry, pastoral ministering, and church leadership. Three of the weekends are just for the nurses and include the original five roles of the parish nurse.

Presently there are parish nurse programs in forty congregations in the Kentuckiana area; three of these churches provide their nurses with a salary. It is hoped that as more is learned and experienced from this ministry more churches will make parish nurses permanent salaried members of their staffs.

It has been a privilege to be a part of the parish nurse ministry in the Kentuckiana area for the past eight years. God has blessed this area with very dedicated and caring nurses, and I am grateful for having been called to serve in this special ministry.

Gerri McDaniel: Parish Nursing in the Roanoke Valley

My first experience with parish nursing came in 1996 through the Virginia Baptist Nursing Fellowship (VBNF). The VBNF is an arm of the Woman's Missionary Union of Virginia (WMUV). Jointly we adopted parish nursing as a project. I heard about an eight-day Ecumenical Parish Nurse Preparation Institute sponsored by Shenandoah University. I was anxious about attending an ecumenical program and asked my Sunday school class to pray for me. I did not want other faiths to influence me. I returned to report their prayers had not been answered, for I had been radically changed. The foundations of my beliefs were the same, but I had experienced God's grace. My walk with God has not been the same since. Previously I had great head knowledge of grace, agape love, and other Christian principles, but I had little heart experience.

The awareness of God's grace and love came to me in a most different manner than in the past. At the parish nurse education program, God began dealing with my legalistic mind. I found other Christian nurses from non-Baptist denominations having beliefs similar to mine. My way was not the only way of seeing God. As we shared during the sessions, I found similarities in our theologies. I also found that having differences in our theology did not negate the similarities or cause me to compromise my theology.

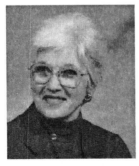

Gerri McDaniel, RN, graduated from Norfolk General Hospital School of Nursing. She holds certification as a nurse administrator and rehabilitation registered nurse. She earned a certificate in parish nursing from the Ecumenical Parish Nurse Training Institute, Shenandoah University, and a pastoral care certificate from Virginia Baptist Hospital. Her current positions include parish nurse coordinator, Women's Missionary Union of Virginia, and Roanoke Valley Baptist Association, coordinator of the Virginia Parish Nurse Education Program, and volunteer parish nurse at Lynn Haven Baptist Church.

As the days passed God confirmed He knew who I was, and that He was the only one who could unravel the weaknesses of my life. He was the only one who knew the whole picture and I trusted Him to show me, day by day, where he needed me to be. Two months after attending the program about parish nursing I became the volunteer WMUV/VBNF parish nurse coordinator. My role took on two parallel pathways: the pathway of education development and the pathway of congregation support.

Pathway of Education Development

The need for education about parish nursing in our area was apparent as we had only a brochure and we were asking nurses to start a program. I felt unqualified to take on development of educational programs. Parish nursing was becoming known, and a substantially qualified collaborative group soon emerged including Sara S. Brown, RN, BS, MDiv; Reverend Donna Coffman, RN, BS, LCSW, MA/DIV; Barbara Huffman, MSN; Judith W. Livesay, BSN; Arranna (Anna) C. McDowell, BSN, RN; Jane Wayland, BSN, MSN; Nancy B. Moore, RN; and myself.

From our collaborative effort the Virginia Parish Nurse Education Program was developed and now provides a quarterly four-weekend continuing education option, and a once-weekly semester college credit option at College of Health Sciences in Roanoke. Ninety nurses representing six denominations have completed these programs. We meet monthly to evaluate and update the program. As a group, the VPNEP decided not to partner our program with the International Parish Nurse Resource Center. Our program included the same basic preparation content plus additional content. Currently, I am the VPNEP chairperson as part of my responsibility as VBNF/WMUV parish nurse coordinator.

Pathway of Congregational Support

The pathway of congregational support developed when in 1997 I became the parish nurse coordinator for the Roanoke Valley Baptist Association (RVBA). In the RVBA we have seventy-two churches. There are thirty volunteer nurses in eighteen of the churches and no paid parish nurses. With the churches I am involved in initiating and starting ministries, development, orientation of nurses and churches, and continual support, networking, health fairs, and some delivery of parish nursing in churches that do not have a parish nurse. Most of the parish nurses have full-time public jobs and families; some can volunteer time only when they are already at church.

The parish nurse ministry is different with each church and nurse. A nurse with experience in adolescent psychiatry has office hours for consultation during the youth group meetings; a nurse with experience in lactation and newborns coordinates a new mom's parish nurse ministry involving the church lay support as well offering her own expertise; a parish nurse connects a person who has just lost a spouse with a qualified church member to help navigate the hospital and insurance process to get bills paid so the person left behind is released of this responsibility and can grieve more effectively; a parish nurse coordinates retired seniors in providing transportation ministry to other seniors who can no longer drive; a parish nurse provides health education, senior aerobics, and health consultation.

In another church, a couple who both worked lost the caregiver of the wife's mother and parish nurses were able to do a needs assessment, provide a plan of care, and mobilize a group of five shut-ins. Each of the shut-ins called this woman one day a week to provide companionship, mostly being a friend by phone and offering reminders to take medicine, eat meals, take a nap, and the time of favorite television programs. The gap was managed and provided the couple time to find an appropriate assisted-living arrangement and prepare the mother for the change.

When the mother was placed in assisted living the five shut-ins who provided telephone reminders called the parish nurses for another assignment. The stories of volunteer parish nurses go on and on.

In most of the churches a vote is taken to adopt the ministry as church-sponsored ministry and the program is added to the church's liability insurance. A commissioning service is held in which the nurse as well as the church commits to this ministry. Even if nothing but blood pressure screenings occur, a statement is still made that the church is about caring for the whole person.

The RVBA parish nurse coordinator position allows me to provide orientation and programs suitable for nurses within my Baptist Association. I work twenty hours a week with a budget including salary and benefits. The WMUV has seen the viability of the parish nurse coordinator position and supports me part time for ten hours a week.

WMUV in conjunction with Virginia Baptist Homes and the Virginia Baptist Resource Center has developed At Home Ministries (AHM). This was developed using the philosophy of parish nursing, and is coordinated by a paid nurse. The mission of the AHM program is to enable churches to assist seniors staying in their homes as long as possible. Information about AHM can be obtained at <www.wmu-va.org> and clicking on the AHM icon. My personal experience in parish nursing and consultation has shown increasing need for seniors' holistic health needs. I find these needs overwhelming for me and our volunteer nurses. Paid staff positions for parish nurses to seniors are needed in our churches. When there is not a specific minister to seniors the pastors are overwhelmed and needs often go unmet. A pastor called me after he took the nurse on his rounds to visit shut-ins and said, "What a burden is lifted from my shoulders, to have a parish nurse who I know will now follow through with the many needs I saw but did not have the time or expertise to address." More information about VPNEP can be found at <www.wmu-va.org>, linking to missions and parish nursing or <www.chs.edu>, linking to continuing education.

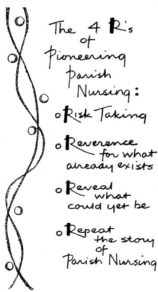

The 4 R's of Pioneering Parish Nursing:

o Risk Taking

o Reverence for what already exists

o Reveal what could yet be

o Repeat the story of Parish Nursing

Dana VanderMey: A West Coast Paid Model

I first heard about the concept of parish nursing in 1986 and felt that God had been "grooming" me all of my nursing career for this special work. I had become a Christian in my last year of nursing school, and had always integrated my faith in my nursing practice. Some of my nursing jobs allowed me the freedom to minister to individual patients' and families' spiritual needs. I always tried to make a point of praying for my patients when prompted to do so. I approached the pastor of our church about the possibility of becoming a parish nurse for our congregation. Although our pastor would have loved to hire me to work full time in that capacity, there were no extra funds in the tight budget. He encouraged me to "hold onto my dream" and see what God would do.

I never lost sight of that dream. In fall 1994, I heard that St. Francis Medical Center was planning to begin a parish nurse program. I applied for the position of director and was hired. I remember being handed the keys to my office and a book on parish nursing, and being told "good luck!" I was expected to begin the program and understood that it would be evaluated at the end of the first year to see if the hospital would continue to sponsor it. Joni Goodnight, whom I consider to be a true pioneer in the field of parish nursing, was hired as a

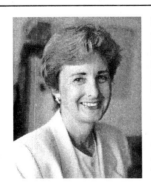

Dana VanderMey, RN, is Director of Volunteers for Hospice of Santa Barbara. She has been a registered nurse for twenty-nine years and brings a variety of experiences to her job. Previously she was the manager of the Congregational HealthCare/Parish Nursing Program at St. Francis Medical Center, Santa Barbara, California, as well as the Liberty Program and the Integrative Medicine Program. She began the parish nursing program at St. Francis and developed it into a national award-winning program, which served as a model and a resource for other communities wanting to start their own health ministry/parish nursing programs. Her nursing career has included years spent as a hospice nurse/case manager with Hospice of Santa Barbara, home health/community health care worker, and critical care nursing. She serves as a deacon in her church and volunteers in various capacities in the church as well as in the community.

consultant to assist and direct me in the planning and implementation phase.

The St. Francis Hospital Foundation committed 100 percent funding for the first year, with the expectation there would be four churches participating by the end of the year. In June 1996, there were twelve participating congregations with five foundation-paid parish nurses serving those churches. The foundation agreed to continue sponsoring the program 100 percent through the third year. The program continued to grow and provide services to the community. In June 1997, the program was awarded the Achievement Citation Award by the Catholic Health Association, a national award given for outstanding community service.

In September 1999 I was asked, along with another of the parish nurses, to do a presentation at the Mayo Clinic during a national nursing symposium. The program was honored locally as well as nationally. At its zenith, the program served twenty-eight congregations represented by ten different denominations, a homeless shelter, Catholic Charities, multiple senior centers, and the like. There were fourteen foundation-paid parish nurses. Some worked full time, some part time, and some per diem. The full-time and part-time nurses got benefits. A nurse had to work at least twenty hours per week to qualify for any kind of benefits. Providing for three churches was considered a full-time position. Most of the churches needed the parish nurse three to five hours per week. We had a three-hour staff meeting once a week, and then there was the documentation, extra health screenings and health fairs, hospital and community events, etc. It was normal for a parish nurse to work thirty-six to forty hours and get full-time benefits. We once tried to assign a parish nurse to four churches, and it was too much.

The foundation agreed to continue 100 percent funding with no restrictions. Then the hospital began to experience severe financial challenges. We were informed that by January 1, 2001, the funding would be cut by 75 percent, and that the parish nursing program would have to become self-sustaining. All the clergy of the participating congregations were invited to a lunch at the hospital where the situation was explained. The clergy were asked to speak to their congregations about covering the cost of their particular parish nurse's salary. The nurses were to remain employees of the medical center with all of their benefits to continue, as well as the support of my supervision. Only eight of the twenty-eight congregations were able to commit to the financial support of their parish nurse. We found grant support for two of the poorest congregations, and we collaborated with Santa Barbara County Public Health Department on a number of community health projects.

I left the director's position to accept the job of Director of Volunteers at Hospice of Santa Barbara. I had thought that I would remain in parish nursing/health ministry until retirement. Unfortunately, the last year in my position was very draining on my body, mind, and spirit. I was required to shift my focus from development and management of the program to fund-raising, grant writing, and begging for money. I am a nurse, not a professional fund-raiser, and I found myself very unsuccessful in the position. As I look back over the past six and one-half years, I think I would have handled the financial support of the program completely differently. I would not have been so complacent in thinking that the hospital foundation would continue funding at 100 percent forever.

We were the community outreach arm of the medical center, and requests for speakers bureau, participation in community health fairs, etc., all seemed to be "directed" to and through our program. Each parish nurse did monthly blood pressure screenings in his or her church, along with other screenings on an as-needed basis. When our screenings revealed individuals without a payment source who needed to be referred for medical care, our hospital was willing to take them all. For the churches it was great when it was all gratis, but there was no real "buy-in." When it came to being asked to contribute financially, money was not available.

Collaboration, networking, toppling barriers, and helping all individuals to access health care is a lofty, but necessary, goal. The faith communities will need to step up to the plate and make a contribution toward changing our health care system through health ministry.

PARISH NURSING IN THE NEW MILLENNIUM

Resource allocation and end-of-life issues will stimulate new roles for parish nurses of the future. "Americans are going to face an immense health care crisis within the next 20 years," says Dr. Harold G. Koenig, known for his research on the role of religion in health:

The population aged 65 and older is simply growing exponentially. Hospitals and nursing homes are already at capacity in this country and we have a shortage of caregivers. We need to examine ways of handling this situation in order to be prepared for what lies ahead, and we need to begin today.[18]

Expectations of parish nurse programs of the future will refocus. The bioethical issues facing older people and their families will require a commitment on the part of the faith communities to become informed from both a theological and a social context. When we speak of care of the elderly in the community the larger picture is the care of families. While caring congregations may provide parish nurses, programs of visitation, and services to homes where an elder is being cared for, it is the family system that becomes the client. Family assessments, leading to addressing health needs of all family members, are a reality that may contribute to early detection of problems.

SUMMARY

The relationship of nurse entry into practice and parish nurse education is an important piece of information for leadership committees in congregations when considering a ministry of health such as parish nursing. For instance, when search committee members look for a director of music ministry, do they want to consider someone qualified to sing in choirs, or someone professionally trained in leading a program of music ministry? The role of the nurse will vary depending on the objectives and motivations of the congregation in which the parish nurse practices. Parish nurse ministry sponsored by a local congregation is complex due to the influences and contingencies external to the congregation. A health minister does not have to be a registered nurse, but for those who are registered nurses, there can be varied levels of educational preparation. Some registered nurses by educational preparation will be better qualified than others to serve as a health minister. The rising number of elderly in the new millennium will, by default, refocus parish nurse ministry as well as qualifications for practice.

NOTES

1. Granger Westberg, "A Personal Historical Perspective of Whole Person Health and the Congregation." In Phyllis Ann Solari-Twadell and Mary Ann McDermott (Eds.), *Parish Nursing: Promoting Whole Person Health Within Faith Communities* (Thousand Oaks, CA: Sage, 1999), pp. 35-41.

2. David Zersen, "Parish Nursing: 20th Century Fad?" *Journal of Christian Nursing,* 1994, 11(2): 19-21.

3. Granger Westberg, "A Historical Perspective: Wholistic Health and the Parish Nurse." In Ann Solari-Twadell, Anne Marie Djupe, and Mary Ann McDermott (Eds.), *Parish Nursing: The Developing Practice* (Park Ridge, IL: The National Parish Nurse Resource Center, 1990), p. 33.

4. Health Ministries Association, Inc., and American Nurses Association, *Scope and Standards of Parish Nursing Practice* (Washington, DC: American Nurses Publishing, 1998).

5. Ibid., p. 7.

6. Mary Ann McDermott, Ann Solari-Twadell, and Rosemary Matheus, "Promoting Quality Education for the Parish Nurse and the Parish Nurse Coordinator," *Nursing Health Care Perspective,* 1998, 19(1): 4-6.

7. Linda A. Jacobs, Mary J. DiMattio, Tammi L. Bishop, and Sheldon D. Fields, "The Baccalaureate Degree in Nursing as an Entry Level Requirement for Professional Nursing Practice," *Journal of Professional Nursing,* 1998, 14(4): 225-233.

8. Editor (1999). "Nursing As a Career," *Nursing Spectrum* [online]. Available: <www.nursingspectrum.com/considernursing/nursingasacareer/index.htm/>.

9. Joanne D. Hess, "Education for Entry into Practice: An Ethical Perspective," *Journal of Professional Nursing,* 1996, 12(5): 289-296.

10. Ellen J. Hahn, Rosemary Bryant, Ann Peden, Kay L. Robinson, and Carolyn A. Williams, "Entry into Community Based Nursing Practice: Perceptions of Prospective Employers," *Journal of Professional Nursing,* 1998, 14(5): 305-313.

11. Jane M. King, Jane A. Lakin, and Jan Streipe, "Coalition Building Between Public Health Nurses and Parish Nurses," *Journal of Nursing Administration,* 1993, 23(2): 27-31.

12. Myron B. Stern and Nicole M. Spring (1999). "Nurse Abuse? Couldn't Be!" *Nurse Advocate* [online]. Available: <www.nurseadvocate.org/nurseabuse.html> Accessed December 4, 2002.

13. E. O. Bevis. "Teaching and Learning." In E.O. Bevis and J. Watson (Eds.), *Toward a Caring Curriculum: A New Pedagogy for Nursing* (New York: NLN Press, 1990), pp. 153-187; Vivian Yong, "Doing Clinical": The Lived Experience of Nursing Students," Contemporary Nurse, 1996, 5(2): 73-79.

14. Kathy B. Wright, "Professional, Ethical, and Legal Implications for Spiritual Care in Nursing," *Image,* 1998, 30(1): 81-83.

15. Elizabeth Bethune and Sally Wellard, "The Commodification of Specialty Nurse Education," *Contemporary Nurse,* 1997, 6(3-4): 104-109.

16. Sybil D. Smith, "Response to God's Life-Giving Ways by Ralph Underwood" *Insights, Austin Seminary Faculty Journal,* 1999, 114(2): 29-32.

17. Ibid.

18. Harold G. Koenig, (2001). <http://dukemednews.duke.edu/news/article. php?id=32>. Acc`essed December 4, 2002.

PART II:
SEEKING STRUCTURE

Chapter 5

Models for Congregational and Parish Nursing Programs

Sybil D. Smith

In this chapter three models for viewing parish nurse programs are presented. The models slowly came to light for me over a period of several years. I struggled constantly with living in the now of providing education and resource support for a large, volunteer parish nurse network, and pulling back from daily tasks to make some meaning of where it all fit into a bigger picture. In 1999, I was asked by the editor of *Insights* to review Dr. Ralph Underwood's well-expressed paper on healing and wholeness, and to write a response from a nurse's view.[1] The opportunity allowed my internal reflections to metamorphose into my initial written thoughts on three ways to view parish nursing: mission/ministry approaches, marketplace approaches, and access approaches.[2] In subsequent publications I continued to expand the way of thinking about parish nursing.[3,4,5] Without understanding the underlying assumptions behind parish nurse programs, it is impossible to evaluate what is taking place. As pondered in Chapter 2 of this book, whose objective is the program trying to meet? It is also difficult to evaluate program effectiveness when the targets of program interventions are not clearly planned or articulated. Intervention strategies for parish nurse programs are also introduced.

THREE MODELS

Three models are presented for the purpose of offering information to church leaders who are involved in decision making about the type of parish nurse program that would best complement the mission of their churches. Each model represents a different philosophy and has specific underlying assumptions. In many programs the models overlap.

Mission/Ministry Model

In the mission/ministry model of parish nursing, the nurse can be unpaid or paid staff on the ministry team of the congregation. Members of the congregation are served by a nurse from inside their own congregation. The nurse discerns a spiritual call to congregation care ministry. The focus is not on the role of the nurse but on persons served. The mission/ministry model relates that in answering the call to be a steward of the faith, one finds purpose and meaning in professional ministry on behalf of personal faith, either paid or unpaid. Faith formation is at the core of congregations and it is within faith formation that one can come to understand the integration of faith and health.

As the nurses practicing from this model are personally finding meaning and purpose in the ministry of congregational care, they come together in worship and prayer with the persons to whom they minister. In Christian solidarity and member-focused care the parish nurses find and can share the healing ministry of Jesus in the congregation where God's word is proclaimed, sins are confessed and forgiven, and the ordinances or sacraments are practiced in fellowship with Christians.

Mission answers the "why" and ministry answers the "what."[6] Authority comes from being called by God to ministry, and becoming endorsed or installed by the congregation to perform that ministry as it complements the larger mission of the congregation. The parish nurse serves the congregation at the pleasure of the pastor, board, or organizational structure, and for the purposes defined by the ministry plan of the congregation. Objectives of the parish nurse ministry are directed by the ministry goals of the congregation through designated process and structure (see Table 5.1).

The journey of faith could be considered the journey to health, healing, and wholeness as it embraces the ministry of reconciliation and integrates faith and health with the driving force of love.[7] Wholeness is considered to be shalom wholeness or being at peace and in harmony in all relationships and situations.

TABLE 5.1. Assumptions of the Models

Assumption	Mission-Ministry Model	Marketplace Model	Access Model
Task	Ministry of reconciliation, health, healing and wholeness, process of discipleship	Offers a commodity, service	Redistribution, emancipation, getting legislation passed. Community process
View of community	Defined by parish	Social problems that need to be solved	System of privileges
Change strategy	Inside to outside Spiritual transformation	Outside to inside, with information and resources persons will make good decisions	Know the enemy or oppressor and organize to exert pressure. Dilute authority
Role of parish nurse or health minister	Steward of the faith Enabler Independent practice*	Technical expert, mobilizes resources	Activist/advocate Community/public health nurse, advanced practice
Power structure	Parish leadership	Sponsoring agency Agency to whom outcomes are reported	Political
Boundary	Defined by parish	Total community or segment, e.g., persons with mental illness	Deprived segments
Conception of client	Parishioner or parish designated	Consumer	Victims/oppressed
Program evaluation	Transformation	Entitlement Utilization focus	Empowerment

Source: Sybil D. Smith, 1998.
*ANA/HMA Standards of Parish Nurse Practice

Marketplace Models

Marketplace models of parish nursing are usually connected in some way to health care systems, operating through home health, case management, community outreach, or other departments within a health or hospital system. Marketplace programs are driven by economic values and offer a commodity to a congregation. Sometimes they are a marketing or public relations tool. The church building becomes the site for delivery of health services.

Positions are paid. The nurse may or may not be a member of the congregation. Often the nurses, with knowledge of community health nursing concepts, are employed by collaboratives or partnerships, and are technical experts in the mobilization of resources for church members. The nurse gathers data about what the consumer wants or needs, implements programs, and interacts with bureaucracies.

A nurse may live out personal faith while practicing in a marketplace program, but the underlying mission or "why" of the program has to do with the business of the employing organization. The business side of health care offers a product to a faith community and strives to be culturally sensitive. Since the efforts in some way contribute to the bottom line of a health system, authority is determined in a negotiated arrangement between a congregation and a health system. Marketplace models can offer inreach programs for church members or outreach to underserved geographic neighbors of the sponsoring congregation.

Accountability in marketplace models is to the health system or funding agency. Some health systems offer services to congregations at no cost, but expect a photo option or publicity for their efforts, and others negotiate a fee to be paid by the congregation to the health system for the provision of a nurse, chaplain, or specific program. Congregations can become involved in marketplace models in an effort to find a way to pay their parish nurse.[8] Often these programs impose strict standards for quantitative outcomes.[9] Although persons may be served well by marketplace programs, marketplace programs may not be congruent with a congregation's ministry goals if the leadership of the congregation feels ministry should originate from within the congregation. In some faith traditions it would be inappropriate to impose external regulations on the ministry of the congregation.

The community is viewed as a system of consumers with social problems that are to be solved by experts. The substance may be tied to a community indicator, such as high incidence of heart disease, or it could be on a calendar schedule, such as a different emphasis each month such as heart month, diabetes month, etc. The consumers can be individuals in congregations who want health programs on site, such as congregation groups that want to financially support a nurse to provide for the underserved; or partnerships and collaboratives that want to improve access to health care (see Table 5.1).

Access Models

Access models of parish nursing are driven by community development theories of advocacy, poverty, justice, and empowerment, and are often tied to philosophies of public health science and community health believing in equal access to health care. The programs are political in nature based on equal access for all resources and aim to realign existing resources between a dominant culture and the oppressed.[10] Positions are paid or unpaid. Often access programs are part of community coalitions. Faith can be expressed through access models as some will offer programs to instill hope and teach that having a future is found in delaying gratification. Access models emerged in response to the decline in accessible health care services, as government organizations began to seek community partners to assist with responsibilities of meeting the health care needs of our poor.[11]

The nurse is an advanced practice nurse specialized in community health and public health nursing. Knowledge of working with aggregates and capacity building is essential. As an advocate for the oppressed, the nurse is a catalyst or change agent to promote empowerment outcomes. The nurse as a social change agent may or may not fit into the ministry plan of a congregation. Some faith communities promote social justice more than others.

Substance is developed from a generosity of spirit and a commitment to social justice. Generosity of spirit is an ability to acknowledge an interconnectedness—one's debts to society—that binds one to others.[12] The call is action based for a common good that leads to changes in the relationship between our government and our economy. Program-level goals in this model seek to influence the political process and contribute to the recovery of social ecology. Individual-level goals revolve around helping the oppressed populations become self-sufficient and engage in some way with a sense of direction for their own life. Attempts are made to break the downward spiral and hopelessness in oppressed and marginalized groups. Problem-posing education methods are valued since they affirm persons as beings in the process of becoming (see Table 5.1).[13]

Summary of Three Models for Parish Nursing

It is important to point out that the writer has laid out discrete extremes where, as in actual practice, there is much overlap. Hopefully these insights will contribute to improved methods of program evaluation for health ministries. These three models are offered as a theoretical lens from which the parish nurse, parish pastor, and chaplain can seek to clarify their aims and purposes in coming together for a health ministry. In the mission/ministry model, the conception of the client population is the individuals and families served by the faith, and the power structure is the parish leadership. The marketplace model provides a commodity to a consumer with the power structure being the agency to which the nurse or chaplain report outcomes, suggesting congregation leadership should enter with eyes open. In the access model services are provided to victims of society and the power structure is political. Ministry goals of a congregation may not always be compatible with the visions of a health system or a community coalition.

Many programs exist as combinations of these models and all three models contribute to redefining health. The average person is not aware of the varying differences in philosophy behind parish nurse programs and, needless to say, would not recognize more than wonderful and needed services being rendered. All of the models are usually classified by health systems as some form of community outreach. However, it is the underlying philosophy that will dictate the substance of the programs. In the managed care marketplace, prevention of illness holds the key for improving the bottom line of health care systems, and churches are a venue. Parish nursing as a subspecialty of a professional discipline continues to emerge as a grassroots movement. Yet holistic congregational care has been central to the Christian church since its inception.

Even though mission/ministry models are less popular compared to marketplace models, it is the mission/ministry model that can best respond to existential illnesses. Society has redefined parish nursing from its original Westberg model. Identifying the operating philosophy behind various parish nursing models can help congregational leadership make decisions for a model that is congruent with their ministry goals. Understanding levels of intervention will also contribute to wise decision making about parish nurse programs.

LEVELS OF INTERVENTION
FOR PARISH NURSE PROGRAMS

Parish nurse programs can provide interventions at the individual, family, and community levels in concert with the local congregational ministry plan. Currently, much emphasis is on health promotion, education, healing, and wholeness at the individual level. Although individuals make up families, and families make up communities, the family system as well as the community is in need of health promotion, healing, and wholeness. The consequences of poor family system health and poor community health practices on society are detailed in the newspapers every day as our nation seems to have widespread tolerance of violence.[14]

Individuals As Targets of Parish Nurse Interventions

Individuals have traditionally been the target of parish nurse interventions, with the parish nurse functioning in the roles of educator, counselor, referral agent, and advocate/facilitator to instill faith, hope, and values. Based on assessed needs, usual parish nurse interventions include classes and programs for cardiopulmonary resuscitation, weight control, advanced directives, grief, stress reduction, support groups, and care for the caregiver, to name a few. Many of the programs invite persons to make a lifestyle change. Change is spiritual in nature as persons give up old ways and commit to new ways of living. Spiritual caregiving and support of individuals during times of change is a vital role of the parish nurse. While some interventions overlap into family issues and the parish nurse certainly views individuals in the context of family, it is not the same as the family system being the target of parish nurse interventions. It is not the purpose here to dwell on interventions at the individual level since interventions at the individual level are at the core of parish nursing (see Box 5.1).

Family Systems As Targets of Parish Nurse Interventions

Many family systems are hurting and in need of spiritual care. They must handle changing conditions and extraordinary pressures with fewer supports than in years past. Families are smaller, with fewer able adults available to give care to the youngest and oldest members and to those with special needs. Real family income has in-

---

BOX 5.1. Individual-Level Intervention Strategies

Screenings (blood pressure,   Advanced directives
  blood sugar, etc.)   Support groups
Diet   Other risk-taking behavior prevention
Exercise   Literacy programs
Smoking, drinking cessation   Counseling
Relaxation

---

creased only slightly in the past two decades, while expenses have risen considerably. Economic needs require adults to be out of the home for long periods each day or even to work far away from home. Male-female relationships are often strained. Discrimination by age, race, gender, and disability creates exceptional burdens for many families. Neighbors often change, and families frequently have a weak sense of community. Many families struggle to manage daily stressors with few supports. Some families are isolated and alone. When families falter, everyone suffers, especially the young, the old, and those with special needs. The costs appear as preventable illnesses, deficiencies at school and in the workplace, violence, mental illness, and economic dependency.

Families are in or near crisis.[15] They cannot do all that is expected of them. *Churches cannot assume that all families will protect and nurture their members at all times.* Individual spiritual commitments to value the sanctity of human life and the family are constantly being challenged. Domestic violence is at an all time high. Families need help to resist violence and deprivation within their own homes. Programs that offer interventions for victims and perpetrators of domestic violence are numerous, but there are few interventions for the prevention of domestic violence before it happens. Programs that contribute to the prevention of domestic violence are educative in nature and require a commitment from the entire ministry team. The goal for family support is to reduce the propensity for violence by increasing the protective forces in the home before there is a victim or perpetrator. Young parents today who make a spiritual commitment to value human life and the family may not be equipped with knowledge about parenting and family life. A lack of knowledge about parenting coupled with stressors of daily living create a potential for domestic violence. Persons often need help to increase social skills and the capacity to feel and show care.

Suggested programs that can be offered or coordinated by a parish nurse program for family strengthening throughout family life cycle development are described in Box 5.2. Just as individual-level wellness-promotion programs invite people to lifestyle change, wellness promotion for families begs an invitation and commitment to the sanctity of human life and the family. The church ministry team needs to first commit to family-support programs as a means of supporting sanctity of human life and the family. The role of the parish nurse on the ministry team that makes such a commitment is emerging. It is likely the role will emerge in relation to the parish nurse's academic preparation. Typically the generalist nurse at the baccalaureate level will conceptualize the family as context and the specialist nurse will conceptualize the family as the unit of care.[16]

BOX 5.2. Family-Level Intervention Strategies

- *Preparation for parenthood:* Education about dating, marriage, sexuality, pregnancy, parenting; prenatal classes

- *Families with young children:* Education about infancy, early childhood; new parent education, fathering education

- *Families with school-age children:* Education about childhood, parenting this age; teach parents about being involved in school; homework assistance

- *Families with adolescents:* Education of parents and teens about family life; preparation for teens to live independently; parental involvement in school

- *Families with adult children:* Education about preparing for life transitions; grandparenting

- *Families providing for elderly:* Education about caregiving; education about nursing home placement

- *Families in transition:* Education about death and loss, divorce, remarriage, relocation, stepfamilies, etc.

- *Other services:* Cooking classes; home visitation, births, deaths, etc.; family dinners for specific family education; sanctity of family life education

Family-systems nursing focuses on both the individual and family simultaneously. Some functions include educator about family life, family communications, family counseling, assessing family functioning, family mediation, and a facilitator of relationship building. Faith communities can also extend family-support programs outside the walls of the local congregation into the immediate geographical community.

The Parish Nurse and Primary Prevention in the Community

When extending family-support work outside the walls of the church into the community, the goal is to strengthen the community by strengthening its families. Outside the church walls, the possibility exists for the target families to be of beliefs and attitudes that are not congruent with the beliefs of sanctity of human life and the family held within the church. Parenting curricula based in instrumental learning and involving acquisition of information and skill development may work well inside the church among persons of common belief, but are questionable outside the church. Parents frequently cannot learn new parenting behaviors unless beliefs and attitudes that support old ways of behaving undergo change. Development as a parent depends on the acquisition of new skills and the enhanced understanding of the influences on one's current parenting style.[17] The invitation to change a current style of parenting may best be presented in a created context for change. Mentoring relationships, contextual support, sharing of life experiences, personal beliefs, and alternative ways become the basis for parents outside a faith community to develop realizable options to difficult problems in the home.

Family-support ministries represent a major outreach ministry program for a church in its immediate geographical community. A significant role for the parish nurse when the church ministry team comes to value a family-support program would be the education and coordination of the church volunteers who would be working as mentors with the families in the community. The parish nurse would be a likely link for the family to formal community resources. Formal community resources to address at-risk families are fragmented along many lines, such as (1) target populations—social services, mental health services, criminal justice, etc.; (2) issue—child protection, people with disabilities, criminal sexual assault, etc.; and (3) organizational auspices—

public, nonprofit, county, state, etc. Community response systems tend to be reactive, investigative, coercive, focused on the individual and not the family as a whole, and fail to address spiritual distress. Teaching lay volunteers to navigate and advocate for a family among the formal agencies in a community is pivotal for a strong family support initiative.

Crisis intervention ministries provide emergency food, shelters, and clothing in time of need, but family and community interventions need to begin as violence prevention strategies. The church ministry team, through a family-support initiative in the community, invites families into a belief system that supports the sanctity of human life and the family. An ongoing reinforcing factor for families that commit to change is the presence of the parish nurse. Protection for families occurs through people who care. If spirituality is seen as embracing the whole of what it means to be human, then the essence of spiritual care outcomes is not doctrine or dogma but the fundamental human capacity to enter into the world of another and respond with feeling—the art of pastoral listening (see Box 5.3).

SUMMARY

Multilevel intervention strategies for parish nurse programs have been presented. Individual-level interventions focus on wholeness of persons in the context of family. Family-system intervention strategies place the parish nurse in a collaborative role with the ministry

---

BOX 5.3. Community-Level Intervention Strategies

Antibullying campaigns

Extending individual and family strategies to unchurched families in community

Extending individual and family strategies to underprivileged neighborhoods

Safety education

Neighborhood watch programs

After-school programs for latch-key children

Neighborhood center

Lighting

Respite

Transportation

Community recreation activity

team committed to a focus on wellness promotion for families, enabling them to fulfill their protective and nurturing responsibilities. Among strategies to promote community wholeness is the provision of services that strengthen and support the families of a community. Understanding the various assumptions underlying parish nursing programs and the intervention options for ministry is helpful in creating solid structure for parish nurse programs.

NOTES

1. Ralph Underwood, "God's Life-Giving Ways," *Insights, Austin Seminary Faculty Journal,* 1999, 114(2): 3-16.

2. Sybil D. Smith, "Response to God's Life-Giving Ways by Ralph Underwood," *Insights, Austin Seminary Faculty Journal,* 1999, 114(2): 29-32.

3. Sybil D. Smith, "Parish Nursing: A Call to Integrity," *Journal of Christian Nursing,* 2000, 17(1): 18-20.

4. Sybil D. Smith, "Theoretical Models of Parish Nursing, Chaplains, and Parish Clergy Interdisciplinary Relationships." In Larry VandeCreek and Susan Mooney (Eds.), *Navigating the Maze of Professional Relationships: Parish Nurses, Health Care Chaplains, and Community Clergy* (Binghamton, NY: The Haworth Press, Inc., 2003), pp. 217-226.

5. Sybil D. Smith, "Practice Models and Educational Pathways for Parish Nursing," *Oates Journal* 3 [online]. Available: <http://www.oates.org/joural/mbr/vol-03-2000/articles/s_smith-01.html>.

6. Lynda W. Miller, "Nursing Through the Lens of Faith: A Conceptual Model," *Journal of Christian Nursing,* 1997, 14(1): 17-21.

7. Kenneth L. Bakken, *The Call to Wholeness: Health As a Spiritual Journey* (New York: Crossroads, 1987); Richard J. Beckmen, *Praying for Healing and Wholeness* (Minneapolis: Augsburg Fortress, 1995).

8. Lorona Schuler, "Parish Nursing Is Ministry," *Journal of Christian Nursing,* 2000, 17(1): 23.

9. Renae Schumann, "Collaboration for Mission," *Journal of Christian Nursing,* 2000, 17(1): 22-23.

10. Neil Bracht, *Health Promotion at the Community Level* (Newbury Park, CA: Sage, 1990); Paulo Freire, *Pedagogy of the Oppressed* (New York: Herder and Herder, 1972); John M. Perkins, *Restoring At-Risk Communities: Doing It Together and Doing It Right* (Grand Rapids, MI: Baker House, 1995).

11. Toby Citrin, "Topics of Our Times: Community or Commodity," *American Journal of Public Health,* 1998, 88(3): 351-352.

12. Robert N. Bellah, Richard Madsen, William M. Sullivan, Ann Swidler, and Steven M. Tipton, *Habits of the Heart* (New York: Harper and Row, 1995).

13. Freire, *Pedagogy of the Oppressed.*

14. Arlene B. Andrews, *Promoting Family Safety and Nurture: Steps Toward Preventing Family Violence and Neglect: A Report of the Institute for Families in Society* (Columbia, SC: The University of South Carolina, 1996).

15. U.S. Department of Health and Human Services, *Healthy People 2000: National Health Promotion and Disease Prevention Objectives,* DHHS Public No. PHS 91-50213 (Washington, DC: U.S. Government Printing Office, 1990).

16. Lorraine M. Wright and Maureen Leahey, "Trends in Nursing of Families," *Journal of Advanced Nursing,* 1990, 15: 148-154.

17. Anita Lightburn and Susan P. Kemp, "Family Support Programs: Opportunities for Community Based Practice," *Families in Society: The Journal of Contemporary Human Services,* 1994, 75(1): 16-25.

Chapter 6

Structure for a Church-Based Parish Nurse Ministry

Virginia M. Wepfer
Paul B. Eckel

Pastors are acutely aware of the increasing demands on their time and resources to meet the needs of their aging church members. Examples of these needs are hospital, nursing home, and homebound visits. Help is needed navigating the medical care system; finding assistance in the home, especially for the frail elderly; providing guidance in health and medication concerns; arranging transportation to appointments; and providing support and respite care for caregivers and other family members. A parish nurse, who can speak the language of faith as well as the language of medicine and health, can address these needs.

The development of a parish nurse ministry within a particular Christian church ministry is tied to the chain of decision making in each congregation and can be accomplished using the strategic planning process. This process consists of four major steps: (1) strategic analysis, (2) vision and mission clarification, (3) strategy development and operational plans, and (4) review and evaluation. Strategic analysis will seek answers to What can be done? and Where are we now? In vision and mission clarification the questions, What should be done? and Where should we be going? will be answered. Strategy development and operational plans seek to answer, What will be done? and How shall we get there? Review and evaluation look at, How have we done? and Are we getting there? (See Box 6.1.) The planning process enables the congregation, denomination, or the individual to establish clear and measurable goals. With goals in place

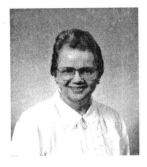

Virginia M. Wepfer, MSN, RN, C, founded, in 1997, Wendan Health Ministries Resource Center, Inc., and is the administrator of the center. She is health ministries coordinator and a parish nurse at the First Presbyterian Church in Warren, Ohio, and has been a parish nurse for six years. She is a certified specialist in staff development and continuing education, has developed and provided programs for parish nurse education, and serves as a facilitator for the development of parish nursing in area congregations. She published *A Parish Nursing Policy Book,* which has gained wide acceptance nationally. Virginia has been the chair of the parish nurse section of Health Ministries Association (HMA) and on the HMA Board from 1998 to 2002. Virginia earned her BSN from the University of Michigan in 1957 and her MSN from the University of Akron in 1983 with a specialty in family health. She is an instructor for the S.T.E.P. program (Systematic Training for Effective Parenting). Prior to involvement with parish nursing, she was a cooperate director of staff development for a national home health agency.

the group can focus its energy in support of the vision and mission. A good set of goals will have the following characteristics:

- Specific
- Measurable
- Achievable
- Realistic
- Time bound

Planning is an important tool for developing a new program because the group goes through the process of establishing its vision and purpose. With a vision and purpose, the goals that are established can be linked and coordinated in a way that permits the new ministry program to be productive and efficient. It is the process of determining direction. The evaluation or control phase ensures that the planning process is continuous, and that the goals will always reflect the true vision and purpose of the congregation and the parish nurse ministry. Planning, therefore, becomes the way to manage. The purpose of planning is to achieve the best possible results, to make things hap-

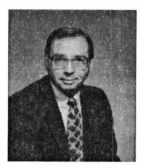 Paul B. Eckel received a master's in hospital administration from Duke University in 1972. He was a health services officer, U.S. Public Health Service, from 1972 to 1977, and was on the faculty of UNC Medical School from 1977 to 1979. Since then he has been a health care management consultant. He works with health care organizations and communities to make health care delivery more available, efficient, and effective. His skill set includes planning, business management, and information analysis. He is an elder in Mitchell Road Presbyterian Church, Greenville, South Carolina.

BOX 6.1. Strategic Planning Process

Strategic Analysis
asks
What can be done? Where are we now?

Vision and Mission Clarification
asks
What should be done? Where should we be going?

Strategy Development and Operational Plans
ask
What will be done? How shall we get there?

Review and Evaluation
asks
How have we done? Are we getting there?

---

pen that would not otherwise occur (Proverbs 16:3). Further, the planning process is helpful to the development of a solid structure for a parish nurse ministry in the following ways:

- Reaching and maintaining agreement on performance and key result areas
- Identifying and evaluating problems and opportunities
- Clarifying goals
- Monitoring important trends that will affect future results
- Gain and maintain support and acceptance

In the various communities of faith, the four planning steps will be addressed in different ways and at different levels within the church organization. The decisions that must be made will fall under the basic planning phases represented by the key questions from each of the four steps in the strategic planning process:

- Where are we now?
- What should be done?
- What will be done?
- How have we done?

WHERE ARE WE NOW?

The vision of the benefits of a parish nurse ministry in the congregation may come from the pastor, a nurse, or other congregation members who are interested in a nursing ministry. A congregation can reap many benefits when a group of interested individuals forms for the purpose of gathering information about the concept of parish nursing. The group effort will facilitate the change process within the congregation. Group members can begin talking about the possibilities of a ministry and gain the support and enthusiasm of others. Numerous resources are available for persons seeking information about parish nursing. A list of a few of the many available resource materials appears at the end of this chapter.

Talking to members in nearby congregations with existing parish nurse programs is a promising source of information. A question group members will be asked frequently is, "What do parish nurses do?" Knowing the difference between medical care (the domain of the physician) and health care (the domain of nursing) is helpful. Even though *Scope and Standards of Parish Nursing Practice* defines what a parish nurse is, each denomination interprets within its framework what a parish nurse does.

Many of the denominational Web sites will identify their views on the contributions of parish nurses to congregational life. The American Baptist Web site lists the following:

What does a parish nurse do?

- Reflects God's love through professional and personal caring behaviors for the congregation.

- Promotes a holistic view of health, integrating body, mind, and spirit within the congregation.
- Works with the ministerial staff in coordinating a health ministry.
- Facilitates the use of community resources.
- Serves as a resource for health information.
- Provides health counseling and referrals for further counseling.
- Promotes and provides health education.
- Encourages health screening and disease detection practices.
- Serves as an advocate for church members concerning health issues.
- Promotes spiritual-based values in making decisions.
- Encourages use of the healing resources of the congregation including prayer, worship, and fellowship.
- Assists with visitation in homes, hospitals, and nursing homes.[1]

Contacts with local hospitals can be made to determine if the local hospital offers any education and resource support for parish nurse ministries. Gathering the information and educating both the laity and the professional staff of the congregation can take six months to a year, or longer.

Identification of decision makers in the congregation is necessary. Decision makers can be provided with resources that will help them make a wise interpretation of gathered information. Endorsement by the pastor is essential.[2] It would not be prudent to proceed if the pastor's support is wavering. A broad base of support is needed within the congregation as well as among the decision makers in the church. Organizational support should come from all levels of the congregation. Answering the question, Where are we now? provides information for the next phase of the decision-making process.

WHAT SHOULD BE DONE?

Once a base of support is evidenced, a formal proposal is prepared for presentation to the decision-making body of the church. The proposal includes a description of the concept of parish nursing and goals of the parish nurse ministry. Goals are to be congruent with the overall ministry objectives for the congregation, complementing the

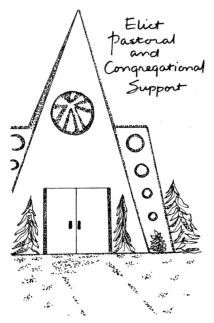

nurturing activities of other, established church groups, such as deacons, elders, Stephens Ministers, etc. Development of the proposal is a joint effort of the pastor and all individuals who gathered information about parish nursing for liability. If the position is to be salaried, a suggested budget is presented with the proposal. If the position is to be one of unpaid staff, a modest budget is included for the purchase of equipment. A sample proposal is included in Box 6.2. Essential requirements for the ministry are a space or desk for the nurse and a locked file cabinet. Liability concerns are often raised during the presentation of the proposal. It is the responsibility of the church to insure the parish nurse ministry for liability. If the presentation is received favorably at all levels of decision making, the establishment of infrastructure can begin.

Development of a Mission, Vision, and Values Statement

Once the concept of, and commitment to, a parish nurse ministry is established, the development of the vision, mission, and values statement for the parish nurse ministry can begin. The process is a joint effort among the parish nurse, the pastor, and other interested individu-

---

BOX 6.2. A Sample Proposal for Initiating a Parish Nurse Program

To: The Ruling Body (deacons, elders) of the (name) Church
From: The Pastor and the Committee exploring parish nurse ministry

The Committee to explore parish nurse ministry, authorized on November 17, 1999, met February 13, 2000. The following recommendations came from that meeting:

1. The church should develop a Parish Nurse Ministry within the congregation.
2. Virginia M. Wepfer, MSN, RN, C, should become a member of the church staff as a parish nurse as of March 1, 2000. A proposed job description is attached.
3. The parish nurse will report to the associate pastor and will make regular reports to the ruling body.
4. A Service of Dedication should be conducted for the parish nurse.
5. The Parish Nurse Ministry should be funded at $500 a month.
6. A request should be made to the Committee on New Ministries to fund the Parish Nurse Ministry through August 31, 2000.
7. Beginning on September 1, 2000, the Parish Nurse Ministry becomes a part of the general budget of the church.
8. The parish nurse will require a space with a desk and a locked file cabinet. Three blood pressure cuffs are currently available. It is envisioned that the library will be used as an area where a nurse can take blood pressures with individual parishioners and also meet with parishioners in a confidential manner.
9. A phone at the desk and access to a computer is requested.

---

als, particularly other nurses. The mission statement for the parish nurse ministry is congruent with the mission statement of the congregation. A good vision statement is limited and focused. The value statement will include key areas from the beliefs of the church, as well as a definition of health and of nursing. Examples of statements developed for a particular congregation are shown in Box 6.3. Development of the statements can generate discussion that clarifies thinking and promotes ownership of the concept of parish nursing for those persons involved in the process.

WHAT WILL BE DONE?

Once the pastor and other church leaders decide to initiate a parish nurse program, an administrative and operational structure needs to

---

BOX 6.3. Mission, Vision, Values of the Ministry

Mission: To promote health and wellness within a Christian faith community using the disciplines of worship, service, and education.

Vision: The provision of a quality parish nurse ministry to all members of the congregation and selected members of the community.

Values related to this parish nurse ministry:

- God lives within the faith community.
- Faith is the belief that God, as revealed in Jesus Christ, cares passionately about our total being: mind, body, and spirit.
- The Holy Spirit empowers the individual to move toward health and wholeness and community members to care for one another.
- Our prayers indicate that the presence and power of God is the abiding force toward health and wholeness that the Bible predicts.
- Health, or wholeness, is the dynamic process of working toward integration of body, mind, and spirit, and toward harmony with oneself, with family and others, and with God. Through Jesus Christ, the healer, we find the meaning and purpose of life.
- *Nursing** is the diagnosis and treatment of human responses and includes the following:
    1. Attention to the full range of human experiences and responses to health and illness without restriction to a problem-focused orientation.
    2. Integration of objective data with knowledge gained from an understanding of the patient's or group's subjective experience.
    3. Application of scientific knowledge to the processes of diagnosis and treatment.
    4. Provision of a caring relationship that facilitates health and healing.

*Source of definition of nursing: American Nurses Association, *Nursing's Social Policy Statement,* 1995, p. 6.

---

be developed through the chain of command of the congregation. At this point the nurse should be hired with the assumption that the nurse will be a paid or unpaid staff member of the congregation, and not a volunteer. As a staff member, the nurse will have a job description, policies to follow, and a single person to report to, usually the pastor. The appendix to this chapter includes a sample job description.

Committee Development

The committee that is formed to gather information and bring the proposal to the church often becomes the formal steering committee for parish nurse ministry. Developing a working committee is as essential as having the support of the pastor. Policies can be proposed for daily operations by the committee and referred to the chain of command for approval. It is helpful to have a representative from each of the various groups in a church on the committee. Committee members can report back to their group about parish nursing activities and plans, and discuss health needs and issues raised by the members. The steering committee will meet frequently for the first three months. There may be eight to ten people on the committee or there may be only two. It is good to schedule the first few meetings when the pastor can attend, so others can see clergy support for the parish nurse ministry. Some churches refer to this group as a health cabinet when most of the members are health professionals.

Meetings at first will consist of educating the members in the concept of parish nursing. Most people are not clear concerning the health promoting, self-care instruction, and other activities a nurse can do without a physician's order. The nurse is responsible for communicating the core beliefs and goals of the ministry. A plan is developed for introducing parish nursing to members of the parish, such as a service of dedication for the nurse and articles in the church's newsletter. The issues now become just how the mission, vision, and values statements of the parish nurse ministry will be implemented in the congregation.

Once decisions are made about the ministry activities to be carried out by the parish nurse program, a plan can be written to determine the path to best reach the goals. By this time in the process, choices have been made and thoughts have gone into the expectations church members have for a parish nurse ministry. For example, if the steering committee has determined that the rising number of elderly in the congregation represents a group with special needs appropriate for parish nurse ministries, what is done next? How does a parish nurse and a steering committee go about executing their intentions to explore parish nurse ministries for the elderly? The example of exploring appropriate ministries for the aging population of the congregation will be used throughout the remainder of the chapter. An assumption is that the nurse is now guiding the committee process.

Assessment of Ministry Needs of Senior Adults

An interview with the pastor is the best place to start an assessment of the needs of the senior adults. The pastor will be able to provide information about many parishioners and describe their needs. The gathered information will identify parishioners who are homebound, have vision or hearing impairments, have no family nearby, have been in the hospital in the past year, have lost a spouse, or are in a nursing home or other special living arrangement. The pastor will probably want the program to start with visits to these parishioners by the parish nurse. Such visits will support the pastor's ministry.

For the next step, a list of the homebound church members can be developed. Other individuals or groups in the congregation that are presently ministering to the homebound in some capacity need to be identified. The role of the parish nurse needs to be perceived as supportive to ongoing ministries, and not give the impression that the parish nurse will take over.

Reverence
for what
already exists

o Ministries

o Organizations

o Outreach
Efforts

o Groups

Policy Considerations

Before initiating a parish nurse visitation ministry, a number of policies need to be developed for the program in addition to personnel policies, scope of practice, and committee policies. There must be a definition of a parishioner or church member, and criteria developed for providing services. Will you limit your services to parishioners only? Will you provide services to relatives of parishioners? How about friends, or community members in general? Policies regarding documentation are needed, as well as policies concerning confidentiality of parishioner information and records, including compliance with the new Health Information Protection and Accountability Act (HIPAA) of 2000. It is prudent to have policies related to scope of practice, medical emergencies in the home, death in the home, safety of the parish nurse, and infectious and communicable diseases. Policy books can be purchased with example policies for parish nurse ministry.[3]

Policy development for the parish nurse ministry should follow the protocol of other groups of the church for policy development. Input from health professionals other than the parish nurse may be helpful. Whatever process is used, developed policies should go through the appropriate channels for a particular congregation, such as a governing board, for approval. Established policy guidelines suggest that all policies be reviewed yearly for continued appropriateness and need for changes and additions. Revisions will need to repeat the approval process.

Parishioners need to be kept informed of the development of the program so they do not forget about it. Minutes of steering committee meetings that include discussions and ideas presented should be widely distributed. Follow-up contacts should be made to find out if people have questions or thoughts about the way the program is developing. A monthly report to the governing body will also keep the program in the minds of the church leadership.

Implementing a Parish Nurse Visitation Ministry

With the support of the pastor and congregation established, the parish nurse position clearly delineated, and policies in place, a health ministry team can be recruited. Volunteer health ministers will need to be educated in the philosophy, goals, and policies of the ministry before making visits. Sample education programs for both groups are presented in Tables 6.1 and 6.2.

A schedule of planned visits should be developed next, completed jointly with all involved if possible. It is best to start small, evaluate frequently, and increase the ministry as time and personnel allow. Decisions need to be made as to who will make the visits and how frequently. For instance, it may be decided that the parish nurse, alternating the next visit with a lay health minister, will see some parishioners. Visits made by others, such as pastors, deacons, and Stephens Ministers also need to be factored in the plan. Nurses of the congregation working in local hospitals may be willing to see parishioners who are hospitalized.

A plan for methods of communicating must be developed and evaluated frequently. There needs to be constant vigilance on the part of the parish nurse to ensure adequate communication between those interacting with parishioners, all the time ensuring parishioner confidentiality. If the parish nurse has a locked box near her desk with a slot in the top, oth-

TABLE 6.1. Parish Nurse Education: Twenty Hours Total, Class and Self-Study

Week	Content
1	*The Healing Ministry of the Church:* The history of parish nursing; the need to reestablish the congregation as the primary focus of health
	Parish Nursing: A Ministry of Health and Wholeness: Definition and application of health and wholeness from a Christian perspective; includes systems theory and family systems theory
2	*Parish Nursing Practice:* Standards of practice for the parish nurse, five roles of the parish nurse, areas of practice, focus of parish nurse-parishioner interactions and communication
3	*Administrative Aspects of Parish Nursing:* Administrative policies and procedures including committees, scope of practice, safety concerns, risk management, legal issues
4	*Nursing Knowledge for the Parish Nurse:* Health behaviors, elements of health promotions; independent nursing interventions, therapeutic communication
5	*Promotion of Spiritual Wellness:* Major spiritual worldviews; a model of the Christian view of health, healing, and wholeness; the mind-body-spirit relationship to health and wholeness; spiritual disciplines; activities related to the nursing diagnosis of spiritual support
6	*Self-Health and Professional Development; Evaluation*

TABLE 6.2. Health Minister Education: Six Hours

Week	Content
1	*Introduction* Historical background Philosophy of health ministries and parish nursing Mission, vision, and values of the ministry
2	*Role of the Parish Nurse*
3	*Role of the Health Minister*
4	*The Parishioner* Interactions; communication
5	*Health Ministry Team* Reporting; data collection Issues of confidentiality
6	*Spiritual Aspects of Health Ministry* Self-development; evaluation

ers can put their documentation in this box. In no case should documentation be placed on the desk or in a mail slot where others may see it.

HOW HAVE WE DONE?

After three months and again at six months and one year, it is time to step back and compare the intended activities with what has actually happened. After the first year, annual evaluations usually suffice. Carefully kept records of events, meetings, and conversations with parishioners make evaluation easier and more meaningful. It is imperative that evaluations occur frequently during the first year to be sure that the parish nurse ministry is headed in a positive direction, and to help all involved remain focused on the mission of the ministry. A review of all steps taken and the outcomes related to discussion and planning by as many involved with the ministry as possible keeps the ministry healthy and growing. Input from parishioners served, as well as input from members of the congregation and leaders needs to be solicited. The focus of the evaluation of parish nursing needs to be on *ministry,* not just on numbers and statistics. Parish nurse programs are a tool to increase the caring community of a congregation and the holistic health awareness of parishioners.[4] A comparison of what can be done, what should be done, what was authorized to be done, and what was intended to be done with what was actually done will reveal opportunities to celebrate the hand of God in the ministry, as well as opportunities for change and challenge.

Evaluation of the Visitation Program

A time and place for a monthly meeting for all health ministers and parish nurses should be established very early. This should include a time of prayer and reflection about the spiritual focus of the ministry, in addition to providing a time for communication and discussion. Feelings about visits made, interactions with parishioners, expected and actual visit outcomes, should all be presented. The focus should be on the growth and spiritual nurturing of each minister, and not simply a report on parishioners or number of interactions. One way to accomplish this is to focus on one aspect at each meeting of the mission, vision, and values statements that were previously developed.

By now, a method for each lay health minister to document a summary of his or her monthly activities should be established, and can be turned in to the parish nurse at this meeting. The coordinator can then generate a summary to present to the pastor and the governing body. For the first few months, the coordinator should present this in person if possible, so that the spiritual aspects are presented and the difference the ministry is making in parishioners lives can be expressed. A careful review of parishioner interactions and parish nurse reflections will lead to the next step of evaluation of the activities of the ministry.

It is not enough to note whether the visitation program works well, or even to develop new methods for smoother operations. The utility of the visitation ministry is directly tied to the depth it meets the needs of the recipients of the ministry. In and out, quick visits to deliver church literature or drop off a casserole are not the purpose for the visitation ministry. Lay health ministers can be trained to assess safety and transportation needs of the homebound. Most likely, other ministry needs of senior adults will be identified and decisions will have to be made regarding appropriateness of response, and possible expansion of parish nurse ministries to senior adults.

SUMMARY

This chapter presented an overview of the strategic planning process as it can contribute to developing solid structure for parish nurse ministries that are congregation based. Not all congregations want an alliance with a local hospital, and the senior adult visitation ministry is a ministry that could be launched and maintained from within the congregation. Other senior adult ministries that could be coordinated by a parish nurse might include respite programs, adaptive equipment loan closets, and transportation ministries.

APPENDIX:
SAMPLE JOB DESCRIPTION FOR A PARISH NURSE

Position Summary: Is a professional nurse and the leader of the parish nurse ministry who promotes the health of a faith community by working with the pastor, associate pastor, other nurses, health ministers, and staff to integrate the theological, psychological, sociological, and physiological perspectives of health and healing into the word, sacrament, and service of the congregation. Provides nursing and health ministry services to identified individuals within the community of faith, in compliance with the Ohio State Nurse Practice Act, the ANA Nursing Standards of Practice, the HMA Standards of Parish Nursing Practice, and the health ministry policies and procedures of the First Presbyterian Church of Warren. These services include health promotion, prevention and counseling, parishioner advocate, facilitator, and the integration of faith and health. Understands that services which require a physician's order are not included in the performance of this position.

Accountable to: The session of the First Presbyterian Church of Warren through the pastor/head of staff

Qualifications: Graduate of an accredited school of nursing and currently licensed in the state of Ohio. Willing to make a commitment to the mission, vision, and values of the ministry. Dedicated to the spiritual growth of self and others; able to integrate own personal spiritual life of worship, Bible study, and prayer into the position. A practitioner prepared or willing to learn to assess the needs of the whole person: psychological, physical, sociological, and spiritual.

Completion of twenty-four hours of initial education for the position plus administrative orientation.

Physical Requirements: Able to use the telephone, and document activities and responses of parishioners. Able to visit parishioners in their homes or in a facility. Has own means of transportation, a valid driver's license, and automobile insurance.

Hours: The parish nurse's hours will vary from week to week; it is expected he or she will average ten hours a week, or 520 hours per fiscal year.

Responsibilities: The various duties of the parish nurse follow.

1. Provides leadership and coordination of parish nurse services to parishioners within the framework of the philosophy and policies of the parish nursing of the First Presbyterian Church of Warren.
2. Works within the guidelines of the current personnel policies and procedures of the First Presbyterian Church of Warren.
3. Actively seeks the input and expertise of the pastors, session, and steering committee.
4. Guides the development of programs and activities to meet the needs of parishioners, parish nurses, and health ministers.
5. Coordinates programmatically the activities of the parish nurse ministry with other related church programs and activities as indicated.
6. Provides for the orientation and ongoing education of parish nurses, health ministers, and others associated with the ministry.
7. Works cooperatively with other members of the parish nurse ministry team and exhibits good communication and problem-solving skills.
8. Maintains a holistic perspective of parishioners, facilitating the integration of faith and health.
9. Acts as a parishioner advocate; assists parishioners to relate to the complex medical care system.
10. Teaches and instructs parishioners in the use of appropriate self-care or health-promoting techniques.
11. Continually evaluates parishioners' responses to interventions in order to determine the progress made toward goal achievement in order to alter the health promotion plan as needed.
12. Is available for meeting with parishioners at the church building or other designated place; is available for telephone consultation by parishioners.

13. May make separate and/or joint visits with pastors to parishioners in their home or in a facility as needed.
14. Ensures that clinical records are maintained according to the guidelines of the health ministry.
15. Ensures the protection of parishioners' rights and maintains confidentiality of all parishioner information in accordance with the parish nurse ministry policies and procedures of the First Presbyterian Church of Warren.
16. Is responsible for ensuring that she or he is free from any health impairments which are a potential risk to parishioners or which might interfere with the performance of this position.
17. Completes at least twenty-four hours of continuing education every two years, preferably pertaining to parish nurse ministry.
18. Directs performance improvement activities of the health ministry.
19. Carries out other duties, responsibilities, and activities appropriate to the position.

Evaluation

The parish nurse's job performance shall be evaluated at least annually prior to the beginning of the fiscal year. At this time, the compensation for the position will be reviewed and modified if necessary.

Recommendation: Carries nursing liability insurance.

Accepted on _____ Signed: _____

Witness: _____

NOTES

1. <www.nationalministries.org/mission/CBM/ParishNurseDoc-A.cfm>. Accessed December 26, 2001.
2. Phyllis Ann Solari-Twadell, "The Emerging Practice of Parish Nursing." In Phyllis Ann Solari-Twadell and Mary Ann McDermott (Eds.), *Parish Nursing Promoting Whole Person Health in Faith Communities* (Thousand Oaks, CA: Sage, 1999), pp. 3-24.

3. Virginia Wepfer, *A Parish Nurse Ministry Policy Book,* Second Edition (Warren, OH: Wendan Health Ministries Resource Center, Inc., 2000).

4. Jan Striepe, *Nurses in Churches: A Manual for Developing Parish Nurse Services and Networks* (Spencer, IA: Iowa Lakes Area Agency on Aging, 1987), p. 25.

RESOURCES

Association of Brethren Caregivers. *Lafiya Guide.* 1-800-323-8039. (Elgin, IL: Author, 1993).

The Catholic [Lutheran, Presbyterian, etc.] Tradition: Religious Beliefs and Health Care Decision. Booklets for multiple denominations and faiths. From the Park Ridge Center for the Study of Health, Faith and Ethics, 211 E. Ontario, Ste 800, Chicago, IL 60611-3215.

Concordia University College of Alberta. *Parish Nursing: A Professional Nursing Education Course.* A ten-week, five-module education course; can also be used in a home-study format. University credit may be obtained. For more information, call 403-479-9348 or e-mail <jporter@concordia.ab.ca>.

Global Ministries of the United Methodist Church. *Health Ministry.* <www.umc.org>. 1-800-305-9857.

Health Ministries Association. *Scope and Standards of Parish Nursing Practice.* 1997. The Practice and Education Committee of the Health Ministries Assoc., Inc. P.O. Box 7187, Atlanta, GA 30357-0187. 1-800-280-9919.

Houts, Peter and Bucher, Julia. 1998. *Helping Families Cope with Illness: A Course for Home Visit Volunteers in How to Be a Problem-Solving Coach.* The Pennsylvania Department of Health: contact on the Internet at <www.hmc.psu.edu/copelink>.

Shelly, Judith A. and Miller, Arlene. 1999. *Called to Care: A Christian Theology of Nursing.* Downers Grove, IL: Intervarsity Press.

Smith, Linda L. 2000. *Called into Healing.* Arvada, CO: HTMS Press. Explores ways to reclaim the legacy of healing within churches and ministry settings. Has an excellent chapter on the origins of Christian healing.

Starting Point: A resource for starting health ministries. From the Carter Center: <www.cartercenter.org>.

Steinke, Peter L. 1996. *Healthy Congregations: A Systems Approach.* Chapters include "Ten Principles of Health," "Promoting Healthy Congregations," "Congregations at Risk," etc. Bethesda, MD: Alban Institute.

Striepe, Jan. *The C.A.R.E. Manual.* A 101-page manual developed to assist parish nurses and health ministers to develop and carry out health ministry. Includes monthly articles that incorporate the use of Abbey Press' "Care Notes," a study section, etc. Health Ministries I.C.A.R.E., 1993. Order by e-mail <hmicare@ncn.net>, attn: Judy Doyel, Pres.

Wepfer, Virginia. *A Parish Nurse Ministry Policy Book.* Wendan Health Ministries Resource Center, Inc., 256 Mahoning Ave, NW, Warren, OH 44483 (Warren, OH: Virginia Wepfer, 1997). Includes such chapters as administrative, committees, scope of practice, infection control, documentation samples, etc. 1-330-654-4517 or <wepfer@neosplice.com>.

Videos

A Call to Wholeness. A twelve-minute video to introduce health ministry and parish nursing. Presbyterian Distribution Services: 1-800-524-2612.

The Healing Team: An Introduction to Health Ministry and Parish Nursing. Twenty-two minutes. Bay Area Health Ministries, 70 West Clay Park, San Francisco, CA 94121. Fax: 415-221-8835.

Chapter 7
Barriers, Difficulties, and Challenges

Carol M. Story

This chapter will address some of the issues nurses confront in the practice of parish nursing. Barriers from within and from without the faith community will be explored. Challenges associated with inter-disciplinary collaboration will also be discussed. Before beginning the discussion of barriers, difficulties, and challenges, the writer will relate her personal journey with parish nursing.

CAROL'S PERSONAL JOURNEY

The thought of combining my faith and my love of nursing in the church as a parish nurse caught my attention soon after I returned to college in 1988 to complete a bachelor's degree in nursing. I entered graduate course work in 1991 and in June 1992 attended a one-week intensive parish nurse continuing education course in Wisconsin. I returned to Washington eager to begin a parish nurse program in my church, but I also had the conviction to begin an educational program for other nurses interested in parish nursing.

While in graduate school, another student, Cheryl Washburn, and I were asked to identify key concepts necessary for a parish nurse continuing education program. Cheryl had also completed a two-day continuing education course for parish nursing and we shared the common goal of developing a curriculum for parish nurse education. We examined sixteen different courses available across the United States, wrote a conceptual framework, and listed the topics we felt were necessary for basic parish nurse education. However, the project was set aside due to circumstances beyond our control.

In 1993 I developed a parish nurse program in my church. I continued to pray that God would give me direction and wisdom about where

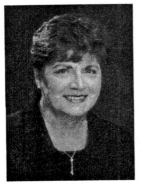

Carol M. Story, MN, BSN, RN, is Program Director of Puget Sound Parish Nurse Ministries in the Pacific Northwest, Seattle, Washington, and serves as coordinator for ministry activities and director of their education course for parish nurses. Carol began the parish nurse network as the first parish nurse coordinator at St. Joseph Hospital in Bellingham, Washington. Ms. Story received an associate degree in nursing from Fresno Community College, Fresno, California, a bachelor of science in nursing from Seattle Pacific University, and a master of nursing from the University of Washington. She is an affiliate faculty member at Pacific Lutheran University in Tacoma, Washington, and former clinical nursing instructor at Seattle Pacific University.

to go with my desire to provide education for nurses called to parish nurse ministry. I struggled with feelings of inadequacy. Cheryl, the only person who knew of my desire to provide parish nurse education, had graduated and accepted a position in Colorado.

Shortly after my graduation in 1993, I was invited to attend a meeting for nurses interested in parish nursing. A few of the nurses had attended a two-day orientation to the concept of parish nursing, but most were at the meeting to learn about parish nursing. When the facilitator of the meeting, Ken Bakken, asked for a volunteer to coordinate future meetings, I was willing.

Five nurses continued to meet on a regular basis and most of the meetings were spent in prayer. One of my early tasks for the group was to meet with and secure speakers for our meetings. In arranging for Chaplain Ray Lester to speak, I was asked to develop an educational course for parish nurses. I looked at him with a blank stare and then shared how God had given me that very goal. Ray said he would write the pastoral care section and he thought Ken Bakken, the founder of St. Luke Health Ministry and Medical Center, a holistic center for patients with chronic pain, would write a section on theology of healing and health. Suddenly, our group had a purpose: to provide education and support for nurses interested in parish nursing.

I decided to move forward and complete development of the curriculum. The curriculum received continuing education approval from

Washington State Nurses Association and we offered the first course in September 1994 for sixty-two contact hours. In 1995, we were invited to affiliate with Pacific Lutheran University, and offered participants the option of college credit or continuing education. In 1996, we registered in the state of Washington as a nonprofit corporation called Puget Sound Parish Nurse Ministries with a six-member board of directors and later received IRS ruling as a 501(c)(3) tax-exempt corporation.

In 1995 I accepted an invitation to facilitate a parish nurse course for the Free Methodist Women's Ministries and I have completed three, thirty-five-hour courses for them. In addition, I have facilitated courses in San Diego, Los Angeles, and Kailua, Hawaii, with a total of 120 nurses completing the same thirty-five-hour course.

I was hired in 1997 as the parish nurse coordinator by St. Joseph Hospital in Bellingham, Washington, to begin a volunteer model of parish nursing. In three years, the network expanded to include fifty-eight nurses in forty-two faith communities. A total of 180 Washington State nurses have completed the class since 1994 to the present. Our data reveal that 100 of these nurses have supportive and viable programs in their church today.

In 1999 our board of directors recognized the potential unfavorable impact of the historical hierarchical structure within nursing, and voted to partner with what was then known as the International Parish Nurse Resource Center of Advocate Health Care (IPNRC) in Chicago. The IPNRC was focused in their continued effort to standardize content and criteria for a core curriculum for the practice of parish nursing. The IPNRC curriculum was then merged into our existing content and continues to be taught by the same ten expert faculty members.

Since 1993 our small interest group of nurses has grown to include a ten-member board of directors, publication of a quarterly newsletter with a distribution of 650, and two annual continuing education days. As I write at the close of 2002, my calendar is nearly full for 2003 with providing weeklong meetings across the United States. I am honored to be a small part of restoring the biblical mission of healing, and I marvel how God works to bring about His purpose in parish nursing, in spite of the obstacles and rubble that fall at our feet.

BARRIERS WITHIN THE FAITH COMMUNITY

To begin a discussion on the barriers, difficulties, and challenges to developing a parish nurse ministry the reader should know that a number of models of health ministry are in place around the world. Important to keep in mind is that every faith community is unique. There are no two programs that "look" the same. I strongly believe that is the way it should be. The variables are different in every congregation. For instance, the mission, the vision, the demographics, the location, the commitment of its members, the history of the congregation, and the understanding of parish nursing, all will affect the outcome of parish nurse ministry.

In my work as a parish nurse coordinator and educator I observe programs at varying stages of development. I walk alongside those who experience the barriers and difficulties described in this chapter. Five barriers from within the faith community are presented.

Barriers Within the Faith Community
Language
Liability Issues
Too Many Church Programs and Not Enough Leaders
Organizational Structure
Job Description and Documentation

Language

A discussion of barriers would not be complete without first mentioning language. This obstacle first became apparent to me when my pastor said three things: (1) "We can't use the term 'parish' nurse, because everyone will think this is a Catholic thing." (2) "People do not come to church to hear about their health." (3) "Holistic health has something to do with new age, doesn't it?" It has been twelve years since that discussion with my former pastor. The same obstacles continue to exist, and the discussion occurs in many denominations. Language both enables and limits our ability to communicate. The extent to which clergy understand the concept of parish nursing will determine the success of the program.

Language barriers can be taken down when both nurses and clergy strive to overcome them by listening to each other, clarifying the terminology used within a particular faith community, and maintaining a teachable spirit, for example, using such terms as *whole-person health* while discussing the interrelationship of the body, mind, and spirit. Facilitating discussion of the rich history of church tradition and its ministry of healing is helpful, as is using the term *parish* as it correctly relates to the geographical location. Understanding how faith and health are interrelated in substance and language ties together the health care system, the health care providers, the values of professional ministry, the congregation, and its culture.

Liability Issues

Questions raised about liability can become problematic if not handled properly. Churches have been concerned with issues of liability for years and there have been lawsuits brought against clergy and the church. In the United States there is a history of lawsuits against health care providers. The role of the parish nurse is to bridge the gap between systems of care and the congregational member rather than to provide invasive procedures.

Even though the risks for a parish nurse lawsuit are low, the responsibility of the church is not negated. The church cannot be lax or negligent in assuring accountability and professional standards are upheld. Nurses, paid or unpaid by the church, will need liability insurance coverage. Licensed professional nurses are held accountable to a higher standard of care than lay volunteers within the church structure. Nurses are accountable to the state licensing board, nursing professional standards of practice, the legal system, and a code of ethics. Morally, ethically, and legally, parish nurses must be accountable for their individual practice. The responsibilities regarding professional liability issues include obtaining coverage for the nurse, reinforcing the professional role of the nurse to the members, and holding the nurse accountable for documentation, licensure, and continuing education within the subspecialty practice of parish nursing. This includes providing funding for liability insurance, funding continuing education meetings and courses, as well as providing physical space within the facility to conduct private consultation and support for congregation members.

Church Responsibilities
Funding Liability Insurance
Funding Educational Meetings and Courses
Providing Physical Space for Private Consultation
Holding Nurses Accountable for Licensure and Documentation

Too Many Church Programs and Not Enough Leaders

Pastors often feel church members are "programmed out," and recruitment of new leaders for new programs can seem like a formidable task. Parish nurse programs arise through the efforts of either the clergy or a nurse who discerns spiritually to develop a ministry of health. It is fundamental to take time to select the right members for the health committee in the beginning and prevent problems later on. Good committee members are those willing to do behind-the-scenes work, those who are not already overcommitted, and a representation from all members of the congregation, across the life span, is vital. It is important to avoid having a committee where all of the members work in health care vocations. Nadine's story in Chapter 1 is an example of not being able to pull together a faithful health committee.

Following preparation for the parish nurse role, the nurse needs the freedom for program development. Program development does not occur overnight. It can take from two to five years for a good program to solidify. Does any volunteer group in a church stay together for that length of time? The church is a fluid organization; people come and go, and volunteers are often overworked. A parish nurse program is started one step at a time. If clergy want to control the management of the program and determine what components it will have, the members will likely not support the program. Likewise, if the nurse comes to the program with an agenda of "fixing" the congregation, the members will likely not support the program. A parish nurse program is successful when the clergy provide freedom for the nurse and health committee to identify the needs of the congregation and together set attainable goals and objectives to meet those needs. Finding the appropriate volunteer health committee members is one piece of the collaborative process.

I was called in to consult with a church that had a health committee in place, eager to begin the program. Soon after my arrival, I learned that not only was the committee all health care employees, but the leader was a semiretired pastor whose role was visitation to the elderly. At a second meeting, some of the committee failed to return and new ones had been added, including the senior pastor who now decided to take charge—and take charge he did. Even though three nurses took the parish nurse preparation course, it was almost two years before the program was up and running because the pastor had to have all the questions answered, everything in place, and all the "ducks in a row" as he saw them, before the nurses could begin. The pastor finally became very well informed and knew and supported the nurses. I suspect the nurses could have done most of what the pastor did, freeing him to the overall church ministry, had he been willing to trust the nurses with the details.

Organizational Structure

Failure of the nurse to recognize that the church functions as an organization can become a barrier. There are politics, differing leadership and behavior styles, communication problems, official and unofficial leaders, and varying strengths and weaknesses within its structure. Knowing one's behavior style, leadership style, and gifts are imperative to success of the program. It is crucial that the nurse understands the history of a particular church: how things are done, how information is communicated, who has the power and authority, and who makes the decisions. When the nurse is not recognized as a member of the staff, miscommunications occur, and the nurse lacks knowledge of how the program fits within the existing structure of the organization.

There can be some negative effects from a nurse practicing in her own congregation that may become barriers to successful programs. The nurse may overextend services because the line between acting as the parish nurse or as a member may become blurred. Members may expect too much, such as late visits, frequent phone calls, and special favors because they know the nurse as a friend and member. The congregation may think the nurse should not be paid because members are expected to volunteer. The nurse may not initiate new ideas because she is used to and part of a system that accepts mediocrity. The role with clergy may be uncomfortable if clergy continues to treat the nurse strictly as a member of the church, and does not accept the professional role. Or the nurse may feel submissive to the clergy as in previous positions working with physicians.

However, the same issues can become positive. The nurse knows the culture and members of the congregation, understands the mission, and recognizes existing needs from participating as an active member.

I was invited to present the concept of parish nursing to a group of ten nurses at a very large church. The pastor had attended a presentation about the concept and had read at least one article on healing and health ministries. At the meeting, his enthusiasm was evident and he asked a number of excellent questions. As often is the case, when I finished the presentation, answered all the questions, and had outlined the role of the parish nurse, there was silence. In the silence the pastor jumped in and said, "That simply seems too overwhelming. We will do our own program." As I looked at the faces of the nurses, I knew immediately there was a dynamic and culture within the church structure that would probably prevent this program from moving ahead any time soon. In fact, three years later, the program was still "what the pastor ordered" and their parish nurse said, "I will do whatever Pastor tells me to do." It is easy to go in with an agenda, become task oriented, and still fail to recognize the needs of the congregation.

During the course of my work, I have learned that nurses need time to process new information, examine their skills, and determine if the role fits with who they are as professionals. Much reflection is needed to balance that information. Parish nursing is not about one person doing things, nor is it about simply having a nurse in the church. It is about transformation and change revolving around the spiritual dimension of the people.

Job Description and Documentation

A barrier can surface when there is no job description for a nurse, or if a job description fails to require documentation of nurse activities. Traditionally, churches do not have job descriptions, and to even suggest that a person should or would document activities that occur within the church brings about comments of surprise, question, and disdain. Without a job description, how can a church hold a nurse accountable? As mentioned in the section on liability, a licensed nurse will always be held to a higher standard of care. Practicing within a church does not change the accountability factor. Services rendered to congregational members deserve the highest standard of care.

A job description not only describes the role of the nurse, but it clarifies the role and eliminates assumptions by members of the congregation and staff as to what the nurse will and will not do. It also establishes a tool for evaluation to determine the success of the program and the effectiveness of the nurse functioning in the role. Further, one job description can lead to the development of others, thereby bringing about positive change and clarification to the meaning of ministry and in understanding staff roles.

State laws require licensed professionals to keep documentation records. Nurses are also mandated to document according to state Nurse Practice Acts and regulations, and according to policies and procedures within the employing institutions. Clergy often accept the explanations, and understand the issues of confidentiality and the need for records.

Difficulties from Without the Faith Community
Education for Parish Nurse Practice
The Meaning of Ministry

DIFFICULTIES FROM WITHOUT THE FAITH COMMUNITY

Difficulties outside the faith community that hinder the development of parish nurse programs are primarily related to two issues. First, education for parish nurse practice is a complex issue and difficult to explain to nonnurses; and second, the meaning of ministry is deeply misunderstood.

Education for Parish Nurse Practice

The former International Parish Nurse Resource Center of Advocate Health Care recommended a BSN as entry into the practice of parish nursing, but also recognized the differentiated practice.[1] At this writing, the most current available data on the breakdown of initial entry into nursing practice of parish nurses is from a 1996 survey of 536 parish nurses in which 46 percent of the parish nurses held only a diploma or associate degree.[2] Data from our Puget Sound Parish Nurse Ministries records of 300 persons completing the parish nurse education course revealed 33 percent held a diploma or associate degree. Data are not available that would correlate viable programs and level of education of the parish nurse.

Parish nursing has been recognized as a subspecialty within nursing, but at this time there is no certification or official recognition of individual nurses as a specialist in parish nursing. In the mid-1990s, rumors were inexhaustible that certification in parish nursing was imminent, compounded by other rumors such as eligibility to write the certification exam would require completion of the IPNRC self-endorsed core curriculum. The misinformation created tension among parish nurses.[3] The national voice for the nursing profession is the American Nurses Association (ANA).

Within the ANA, the American Nurses Credentialing Center (ANCC) accredits state nurses' associations and schools of nursing to offer continuing education for nurses. Providers of continuing education courses for parish nurses submit applications to the ANCC process for approval of the course and authority to issue contact hours. It is reasonable for clergy to expect a credible education program for the parish nurse. Clergy are likely to be more comfortable if the program is hosted by a nursing contingency within their own denomination. Not all denominations provide such support.

Simply stated, a parish nurse must be a registered nurse with a valid license issued by the state in which she or he practices. The wise and prudent parish nurse will not only be licensed but also educationally prepared to function under the guidelines outlined in the *Scope and Standards of Parish Nursing Practice,* as well as the ANA Standards of Nursing Practice. A subspecialty practice would imply one must have additional specific educational preparation. Education from life experiences may also be considered.

The average age of parish nurses is fifty.[4] Implications are that practicing parish nurses in general have an average of twenty years' experience. In addition, years of nursing practice bring expertise, life experience, and wisdom to the role of parish nursing. Therefore, a genuine issue would be, what is the nurse's area of practice and how will that experience and expertise affect the viability and success of the parish nurse program? For instance, a nurse with twenty years' experience as a hospital-based pediatric nurse would need to become

What does "success" look like in Parish Nursing?

current with adult health, community health, and population-focused nursing in general, as well as parish nursing.

In reality, successful parish nurse programs are not necessarily related to level of education but to the individual's spiritual calling and commitment to ministry. This is not to imply that nurses with higher degrees should not become parish nurses. The nurse who has high-quality leadership and communication skills, along with knowledge of community health nursing used concurrently with the call and commitment, will be more likely to develop a solid parish nurse program. From this writer's nine-year observation period of strong, solid parish nurse programs, the key to success has been primarily two factors. First, success has been dependent upon the pastor's support. In addition to the pastor's support, it is imperative that the nurse recognizes that parish nursing is not about tasks and doing things but is about "being with." If the nurse is unable to transition from task orientation to transformation orientation, with the spiritual dimension being central, the program will become just a nurse in the church setting, no different from a nurse in any other setting.

The Meaning of Ministry

The meaning of ministry goes further down the road of educational needs of the nurse. I am continually drawn back to the question: What makes parish nurse practice different from what I practiced for twenty years before becoming a parish nurse? Consultation with clergy in ecumenical, evangelical, and interfaith settings continually reminds me that the single most important ingredient to parish nursing is the spiritual dimension. Clergy want assurance that nurses are bringing balance to the ministry of the church, not just science. Many diverse possibilities exist within parish nursing that are not dependent on nursing. The church is the base of operation with theology providing the conceptual underpinnings for the ministry of the church.

Successful parish nurse programs build on the mission, vision, and strengths of the ministries of the church. Programs are integrated within the natural structure as a whole and thus benefit from the resources and synergy of the entire congregation. To understand and value the meaning of ministry, additional ministry preparation beyond nursing continuing education is recommended for the nurse. Congregations benefit by encouraging and funding the parish nurse's spiritual development via attendance at a school of theology ministry certificate program, and/or through clinical pastoral education (CPE). A host of seminaries offer online courses in health ministry and parish nursing. Many hospitals offer extended units of training in CPE with local congregations being the basis for learning. Spiritual maturity is essential if one is to minister to the human spirit. Ours is a world of suffering and pain, which often draws forth questions about the meaning and purpose of life and opens doors for care of the soul.

CHALLENGES OF INTERDISCIPLINARY COLLABORATION

As a combined term, parish nursing joins two different concepts, church and health. Given this fact, parish nursing is meaningful to both health professionals and ministry professionals. Therein lies the challenge of interdisciplinary collaboration. People who minister within the church do so as members of a pastoral team in which their ministry gifts and professional skills are exercised in close, daily cooperation

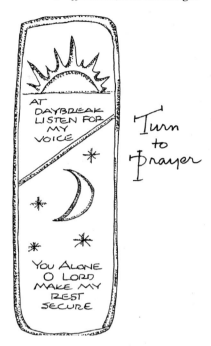

and consultation with other pastoral caregivers. They choose to approach the parish with an explicit commitment to shared responsibility and mutual support in the pastoral care they provide.[5]

Interdisciplinary approaches require a shift from discipline-specific thinking with movement toward integration. Integrated approaches require removal of conceptual boundaries that exist between professions and disciplines. The emphasis is on coordination of specialized knowledge versus dilution of expertise.[6] An interdisciplinary team redistributes the power held by any one member of the team, allowing all professionals to share in the decision-making process.[7] Although the interdisciplinary approach may diffuse power, it does not abrogate individual responsibility, which should be determined jointly.

Ultimately the purpose of collaboration is to foster group cohesion, share ideas, discuss methods of solving problems, and handle conflicts. Interdisciplinary collaboration is a blending of experience and joint knowledge with the potential outcome of new understanding for team members and unity in service to others.

Consider the following case study. A seventy-eight-year-old church member with dementia, recovering from treatment of a hip fracture eight weeks prior, is admitted to a mental health unit. Steps have been taken to declare the member mentally incapable of caring for herself. A petition has been filed by the daughter for protective custody with the goal of placement in a nursing home.

During recovery from the hip fracture, and before the current hospitalization, the church deacon carried communion to the home; the parish nurse made ongoing visits to assure there was continuity of care provided by the daughter, granddaughter, and a sister. In addition to ongoing medical care, the physician was involved in evaluating the mental capacity; the social worker was providing critical evaluation in the ultimate decision made to file for protective custody. The pastor made regular visits to provide spiritual support. Meanwhile, church members provided meals, prayer, and various levels of support in the home. Take away the expertise of any one member of the team of care and what would the outcome be?

The approach calls for a holistic view of the individual in a reciprocal relationship with his or her environment. In other words, people are seen in the context of family and community. The personal interaction, whether nurse, clergy, or other health care provider, impacts the outcome of the person being served. Not only is the impaired church member served but the larger family is also served. Suppose an admission to the nursing home follows the current hospitalization. A new set of ministry needs emerge for the patient and the family members.

Ministry implies collaboration, and collaboration implies teamwork, partnership, alliance, cooperation, and relationship. Can those who work in ministry settle for less than Christ's collaboration with the twelve He sent out as His team to heal the sick, mend the broken-hearted, and minister to the poor in spirit? When ministry teams and others transcend denomination and other differences in faith traditions, they embody a shared vision of wholeness or "shalom" in the true biblical sense.

SUMMARY

This chapter presented five barriers experienced by many parish nurses in the hope of avoiding similar situations in the future. Diffi-

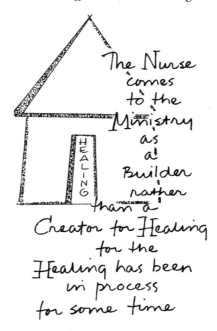

culties surrounding education for parish nurses in the past decade were presented with the challenge to also consider theology course work for parish nurses. Even though we carry many of the same issues into the new millennium, they will be tempered by the rising number of elderly. The rising number of elderly will place demands on congregations that will draw forth the challenges of interdisciplinary collaboration.

NOTES

1. Phyllis Ann Solari-Twadell, "The Emerging Practice of Parish Nursing." In Phyllis Ann Solari-Twadell and Mary Ann McDermott (Eds.), *Parish Nursing: Promoting Whole Person Health in Faith Communities* (Thousand Oaks, CA: Sage, 1999), pp. 3-24.

2. Phyllis Ann Solari-Twadell, "Nurses in Churches: Differentiation in Practice." In Phyllis Ann Solari-Twadell and Mary Ann McDermott (Eds.), *Parish Nursing: Promoting Whole Person Health in Faith Communities* (Thousand Oaks, CA: Sage, 1999), pp. 252-253.

3. Donna Coffman, "My Position on the Endorsed Curriculum at This Time," <http://www.oates.org/journal/mbr/vol-03-2000/articles/s_smith-sb5.html>. Accessed December 8, 2002.

4. Janet K. Kuhn, "A Profile of Parish Nurses," *Journal of Christian Nursing,* 14(1); 1997: 26-28.

5. Joseph T. Kelly, "Five Group Dynamics in Team Ministry," *The Journal of Pastoral Care,* 1994, 48(2): 118-130.

6. Carla Marino, "The Case for Interdisciplinary Collaboration," *Nursing Outlook,* 37(6); 1989: 285-288.

7. Deborah Natvig, "The Role of the Interdisciplinary Team in Using Psychotropic Drugs," *Journal of Psychosocial Nursing,* 29(10); 1991: 3-8.

PART III:
USING THE FEEDBACK

Chapter 8

The Experience of Parish Nursing

Sybil D. Smith

This chapter is not intended to be a discourse on worldviews and religions but does require a little patience for the opening rhetoric in order to make a practical application later on in the discussion. Parish nursing will be discussed in relation to the varied experiences of the nurse, the elements of culture, and how the relationship between faith and health plays out in varying faith groups. The presented narratives from pioneering nurses explicate the variations in practice.

THE CONTEXT OF PARISH NURSING

The experience of parish nursing is unique for each nurse who embraces the concept. Our society and history shape our experience with parish nursing. First, the age when we confront parish nursing is to be considered. The impact of parish nursing in our lives is related to the age when we were first exposed to the concept. Our biological age contextually adds all of the historical events experienced by our birth cohort. Second, we experience parish nursing based on the systems of advantage or disadvantage in our lives. The systems of advantage and disadvantage draw forth our adaptive resources or our capacity for coping with change. Related to our capacity for coping are the opportunity structures available to us as we go through time.

Our age, our experience with systems of advantage and disadvantage, our adaptive resources, and opportunity structures format all of our experiences, not just the experience of parish nursing. Becoming a parish nurse is understanding, at an individual level, where we are in relation to our life experiences. These experiences impact how we view the larger picture of life, as well as influence our actions. Understanding the influence of culture contributes to grasping the bigger picture around us.

ELEMENTS OF CULTURE

According to Daniel Fountain, who extended the original work of Lloyd Kwast, four elements of culture influence what we do.[1] The core of cultural existence is what a society considers to be real. The core is about faith and spiritual foundation and drives our beliefs. Our beliefs in turn drive our values, and our values impact our behavior. Figure 8.1 depicts the four elements of culture: faith, beliefs, values, and behavior. The four elements of culture represent a useful model for understanding the difference between parish nursing as a ministry of transformation, and parish nursing as a vehicle for delivery of biomedical health promotion and prevention education services. Since

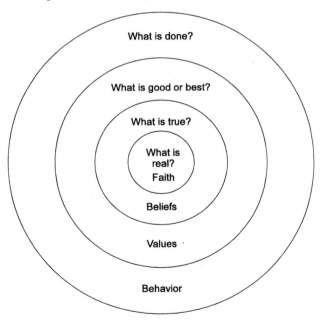

FIGURE 8.1. Elements of Culture (*Source:* Adapted from Lloyd Kwast as used in Dr. Dan Fountain's monograph, *Health, the Bible, and the Church,* and used by permission of the Billy Graham Center, Wheaton, IL 60187-5593, and the William Cary Library, Pasadena, CA.)

parish nursing holds the spiritual dimension to be central, and the focus of parish nurse practice is the faith community and its ministry, it is important to explore the elements of culture and relate them to diversity in parish nurse practice.

Parish nursing is rooted in Christian tradition. Non-Christian faith groups also participate in parish nursing. Since all religions have a point of exclusion it is important to carefully consider Figure 8.1. Even though Chase-Ziolek and Holst report minimal conflicts when providing parish nurse programs across varying religious groups, the larger picture needs to be considered.[2] Most parish nurses work within their own faith community. However some parish nurse programs from a community-development or access model framework do pay parish nurses to work among faith groups not similar to their own. Providing preventive and health promotion services to a congregation is not the same as providing ministry as defined by one's system of faith. For instance, as an extreme example, a faith system may hold to the belief that it is wrong to accept certain medical and surgical interventions. In such a situation there is a potential for conflict when the professionally licensed nurse cannot support the members in being loyal to the belief of the faith system regarding refusal of medical and surgical interventions.

Because faith informs beliefs and values, it defines health and healing for each faith group. A belief system is an outgrowth of the faith system and orders people to live in a certain manner. Persons who do not participate in an organized faith community still confront the question, What is real? All persons wonder where they came from and where they will end up when they die, and search for meaning and purpose in living. The difference is in the substance of the answer, even when persons cannot define the substance. Varied substance exists in the contrast between the sacred and the secular. Faith also dictates our behaviors. Whole-person health is not the same for all faith groups. Not all faith systems accept shalom wholeness as health, yet health is discussed in those terms throughout this text. Not all faith systems value human life equally. In some faith systems values are absolute, and in other faith systems values can be relative. Physical well-being can be more easily understood among diverse groups: either the pieces and parts of our body are working properly or they are in need of an intervention. For instance, most would agree that an open, actively bleeding wound needs an intervention to stop the bleeding. Spiritual well-being will be experienced differently across religious groups. It is tied to beliefs about the source of meaning, purpose, suffering, and destiny. The body of literature is growing to support the relationship between physical and spiritual health. Because of varying systems of faith, parish nurse intervention strategies will vary across the faith systems.

To explain the differences in the intervention strategies, I have borrowed with permission from Daniel Fountain's two descriptions of health education.[3] First is the behavior-oriented approach as shown in Figure 8.2, and then the culture-oriented approach shown in Figure 8.3. The behavior-oriented approach is one I have coined as the outside-to-inside approach to intervention strategies. The culture-oriented approach I have coined as the inside-to-outside approach to interventions. Numerous activities exist for persons to choose from for the promotion of desired health outcomes. The question becomes, What is the motivation required for the activity?

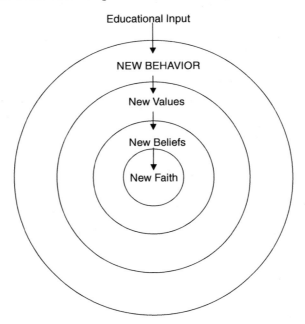

FIGURE 8.2. Behavior-Oriented Education (*Source:* From Dr. Dan Fountain's monograph, *Health, the Bible, and the Church,* and used by permission of the Billy Graham Center, Wheaton, IL 60187-5593.)

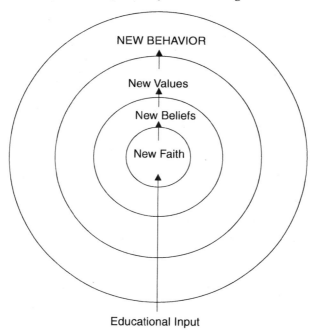

Educational Input

FIGURE 8.3. Culture-Oriented Education (*Source:* From Dr. Dan Fountain's monograph, *Health, the Bible, and the Church,* and used by permission of the Billy Graham Center, Wheaton, IL 60187-5593.)

Outside-to-Inside Approach

The outside-to-inside approach is about following all of the rules to obtain desired outcomes. Following the rules is about acts of the will. In other words, by an act of one's will, a person can choose to eat right, drink right, reduce stress, and avoid harmful substances. Values and beliefs are not the target of the interventions.

As a person's behavior changes by application of the rules and recipes for desired outcomes, it is assumed that the change in behavior will stimulate reflection about values and beliefs. The internalization of an externally imposed restraint will be difficult to accomplish without the simultaneous transmission of values and beliefs. A regimen of things to do and not do can often lead to resistance. The road to changed behaviors that will improve health outcomes from the outside to inside also requires a conducive environment for the approach to be applied.[4]

Inside-to-Outside Approach

The inside-to-outside approach is about an internal transformation which begins with the premise of faith and beliefs. Motivation, when considering an inside-to-outside approach, is tied to loyalty to faith and beliefs. It is about living out one's faith. Individuals must understand their faith before they can assimilate the health-promoting practices of the faith. Once a person understands his or her personal faith and health relationship, he or she can explore making the choices that contribute to desired health outcomes. Even with the knowledge of one's faith system, people do not always make wise choices and therefore live out the consequences of bad decisions. The journey of faith becomes the daily resolution and struggle to make faith-congruent decisions for living.

Decisions for daily living are made in relation to our experiences with systems of advantage and disadvantage, our adaptive resources, and opportunity structures. One of the opportunity structures available to Americans is the opportunity for a system of faith that one can name and claim. Naming and claiming one's faith system can contribute to integration of mind, body, and spirit, achieving whole health even when a cure is not possible. One's belief system can become an adaptive resource for the promotion of health. Parish nurse programs of the past decade contained both outside-to-inside and inside-to-outside strategies for promoting desired health.

THE EXPERIENCES

The experiences of three nurses are presented for consideration. First the story of Betty Crowell, a nurse with eighteen years of hospital-based work. Betty's life was one of limited systems of advantage, but she was able to maximize her adequate exposure to opportunity structures through her adaptive resources.[5] Virginia Wepfer's story follows entry into nursing practice with a BSN in 1957. Very few nurses were entering practice with a BSN in 1957, therefore Virginia experienced an opportunity early in her life not available to all nurses. Last is the experience of Marie Bott, whose journey to congregational ministries is atypical, but particularly relevant. Marie's story is one of adaptive resources.

Betty Crowell's Story

When I reflect on my experiences during eight and a half years as a parish nurse coordinator for a hospital in northeast Florida, I realize that I am a different person from when I began the journey. I feel blessed that I had the challenge of starting parish nursing in our area. God does not always call the prepared, but God always prepares the called. I have always viewed nursing as a vocation, a Christian call to serve. At some level, I always knew I was only to plant the seeds of parish nursing.

On October 26, 1992, I was hired for a three-year commitment as a paid parish nurse to serve in two local parishes, one Catholic, the other Episcopalian. I was familiar with the term *parish nurse* through Nursing Christian Fellowship. At the time, I had been employed by the hospital for eighteen years. I went through several interviews for the position, which included the pastor and rector of the local churches.

I initially was under the hospital department of nursing. My director sent me to a program of orientation to parish nursing at the Parish Nurse Resource Center near Chicago in 1992. I was in constant prayer. Very few understood parish nursing, and having a nurse as a member of the congregation's staff was strange. The role of the parish nurse is based on a nursing model of caring versus the medical model of curing. Parish nursing emphasizes being rather than doing, which

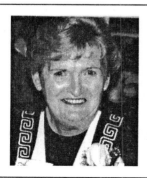

Betty Crowell, RN, BSN, MPS, entered nursing practice in 1957 with a diploma from Holy Name Hospital, Teaneck, New Jersey. In 1985 Betty earned a BSN from the University of North Florida and received a master's in pastoral studies in 1999 from Loyola in New Orleans. Most of her nursing career was in clinical areas until she started a parish nurse program in Jacksonville, Florida, in 1992.

was confusing because we did not do procedures that most people associate with nursing, such as injections, baths, or dressing changes.

I started to use the basic premise of systems theory, that a change in one area will create changes in other areas. The partnering of hospitals with faith communities was another system change, both for the hospital and the participating congregations. Within this precarious balance of changing systems that included health care delivery, the hospital, and the faith communities, I introduced parish nursing. Upon reflection, I realize that within the hospital, nurses are employees, whereas volunteer parish nurses serve their congregations. We were coming from two totally different perspectives. I was between worlds. My answer was to educate the health care system, those who provided care, nursing students, congregations, and clergy.

I developed a mission statement to keep me focused on the purpose of my work. I based my practice of parish nursing on two concepts. First is an understanding of health as wholeness, reflecting the biblical concept of wholeness which is broader than the concept of health as merely physical wellness. Second is the concept of the early Christian communities, especially the Pauline communities, in which members shared their gifts and talents to build up and care for one another.

During this time as parish nurse in the two churches spending approximately twenty hours a week at each, I asked my director if I could start a program to orient local nurses to parish nursing. I asked a nurse educator to assist me in creating an orientation specific to northeast Florida. My main desire was to develop and expand the program. If someone asked me about becoming a parish nurse I wanted to be prepared. At this time, I also realized congregations were not going to pay a nurse because no one in the area was familiar with parish nursing. The program was for those who wanted to be a volunteer in their congregation.

Twelve nurses participated in the first parish nurse orientation, representing several denominations. When the nurses and their congregations wished to participate in parish nursing, I advocated for a covenant relationship with them. A Methodist minister assisted in writing the covenant agreement between the hospital and the congregations. I wanted the covenant to originate from the church rather than the legal department of the hospital. The covenant went back and forth numerous times before being approved.

As the program grew, I realized parish nursing was more than nursing. I changed the title of parish nursing to "ministry" in 1995. I used family system concepts in dealing with congregations, recognizing each congregation as being unique with a distinct interaction style. Many times something would work in one congregation and not in another.

In 1996, I started my master's degree in pastoral studies, with an ecumenical focus (ministry to the world or kingdom ministry), through Loyola University in New Orleans where I defined parish nursing as ministry for my thesis project. I had been working fifty-plus-hour weeks, including Saturdays and Sundays for eight years. My health began failing in January 1998. I thought I might have cancer again and resigned in May 2001. The program is currently stable with fifty-plus congregations, representing twelve denominations, with 250 volunteer registered nurses participating. I am presently a chaplain intern in a clinical pastoral education program.

Virginia Wepfer's Story

I attended an Ohio Nurses Association convention in 1994, and went to a presentation about parish nursing. The concept touched my

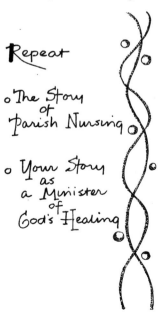

spirit, and I was convinced that this was a ministry I wanted to pursue. My master's degree is in family health nursing and I had been working in the field of home health care for many years, moving from a staff nurse to a staff development educator at the national level. I have been very active in the Presbyterian church all of my life. To me, this background was a perfect fit for parish nursing. I was also deeply concerned about the gaps in our medical system, such as access to a health professional and the fact that the proposed universal health care reform had been defeated.

After a move in 1996, we joined a small rural church. A nurse there had visited with a parish nurse in Columbus, Ohio, had support of the pastor, and had gained the approval of the session (the ruling body of a Presbyterian church) to develop a parish nurse ministry. She and the pastor welcomed my time and expertise. With the enthusiastic support of the pastor, we obtained two grants from the Presbyterian Church, USA: one for the development of the new ministry, and the other for the development of a resource center to promote parish nursing in other churches. The vision we had was to establish a model parish nurse ministry at the church where I would be part of the staff as the health ministry coordinator, and to establish an educational/resource center where I would take the role of administrator and educator. Both of these were paid positions.

This was indeed an exciting time. I resigned from my full-time home health educator position, full of anticipation. I felt called to this vision and this was reaffirmed in the response I received from the pastor, the other parish nurse, members of that congregation, the Presbytery, and from many nurses in the community. The complete structure for our parish nurse ministry was developed and established, and I regularly visited parishioners, taught wellness workshops, and supported the pastor in his ministry. The spiritual rewards of these activities were far beyond my expectations. I always seemed to be at the right place at the right time. I could see the spiritually healing results of joining health concerns with faith, and I experienced deep, personal spiritual growth.

We established the Wendan Health Ministry Resource Center, Inc. I wrote *A Policy Book for Parish Nurses,* and developed and taught a course in parish nursing that awarded 26.6 contact hours for nurses. I attended both the Westberg Symposium in Chicago, sponsored by the

International Parish Nurse Resource Center, and the Health Ministry Association Conference on a yearly basis.

By the spring of 1999, after much hard work over the previous two and a half years, it became obvious that Wendan would not be a self-sustaining entity. It is always difficult when a vision does not become reality. Pastors and nurses in the community would express interest in parish nursing, but the excitement and commitment seemed to be missing, the idea dropped, and Wendan services were not requested. Since the parish nurse ministry at this first church was well established under the direction of the other nurse, I began to look elsewhere for a place to establish another parish nurse ministry. After a number of interviews, in the fall of 1999, the Lord directed me to a 400-member church where both pastors were very receptive to the idea. As one pastor said, "If God has led you to this ministry, who am I to say no?" I met with a nurse from the congregation, who was soon asking, "How are *we* going to do this?" and knew I had met a kindred spirit. She attended the parish nursing classes offered by Wendan and gained knowledge and insight into such a ministry.

In November of 1999, eleven people attended a meeting for those interested in the ministry. Eight agreed to be on a steering committee. I began to place information about parish nursing in the monthly newsletter and the bulletin, and to meet regularly with the associate pastor, who would be guiding the ministry. After a second steering committee meeting in February 2000, work began on a resolution to be presented to our governing body (session) for the ministry with a paid, part-time staff position for me as the health ministries coordinator and parish nurse. The resolution was accepted, a task force began to revise policies in the policy book to fit this congregation, and the personnel committee began work to establish the staff position.

As expected, we met resistance. It was proposed to change the position to a volunteer position on a trial basis, without a full job description. The session withdrew its approval of the resolution, declaring that it was not fully understood at the time. This was a situation in which the knowledge of change theory helped me to deal with the rejection of the concept of parish nursing. With the full support of the pastors, the other nurse, and many in the congregation, education of the congregation continued. With policies in place, I began to provide requested respite care for a parishioner and visit a few other parishioners after the resolution was first accepted; the pastors, steering committee, and I decided that I should continue these activities. I attended as many church functions as possible, and continued to place health information in the newsletter. The pastors, members of the steering committee, and nurses talked to individuals whenever possible to present the concept of parish nursing as a ministry of support to the pastors and a service to the congregation. At their meeting in April, the resolution was again passed by the session. I met with the pastors and the personnel committee to establish my job description and reimbursement, and the ministry was under way.

As predicted by group change theory, after two years parishioners are beginning to grasp and accept the concept of parish nursing. People now come to me regularly with questions or concerns that are within the scope and standards of parish nursing. There is an increase in support and teamwork between the parish nurses, health ministers, and other groups within the church, such as our deacons who also visit the sick and the homebound. A focus of ministry, dedication, commitment, communication, and prayer by many individuals has resulted in the growth of the ministries of health at this church.

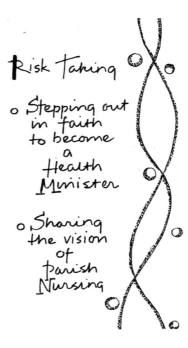

Risk Taking

o Stepping out in faith to become a Health Minister

o Sharing the vision of Parish Nursing

Marie Bott's Story

Sister Marilyn Trowbridge presented a lecture at the Oratory, in Rock Hill. She was the parish nurse coordinator at St. Francis Health System in Greenville, South Carolina. We exchanged names and she sent me more literature about parish nursing. This seemed to be the path that I wanted to follow. Parish nursing sounded like what I wanted to do in my nursing career and service to my church. I was a stay at home mom, but my children were now in school. I worked a half day a week at Hospice Community Care, as needed. Parish nursing sounded like something that would combine my nursing abilities and my spirituality as my hospice work did. I prayed about it and a year went by before I took action.

A friend of mine, Brother Joe Guyon, RN, wanted to take the parish nursing course with me. There were several Catholic parishes in our area and we felt this was where we were being called to serve. We attended the two Saturday orientation classes. I'm not sure what I expected; there was such a deep respect and spirituality in each individual present. The nurses cared about their church families, about nursing, and about making the world a better place to live, starting in their own corner of the world.

Sister Marilyn talked a lot about "planting seeds," but I was already looking to the harvest! Ideas floated through my mind about bringing this to my parish family and what a difference it could make in the lives of those who fell through the cracks of medicine. This often happened because of financial issues, not having an advocate,

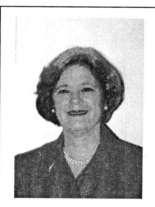

Marie Bott, RN, graduated from Community Medical Center in Scranton, Pennsylvania, in 1975. She has twenty-seven years of experience in the areas of medical/surgical, oncology, cardiology, and cardiac rehab nursing. For the past ten years she has worked in hospice care. Her experience as a cancer survivor has given her firsthand knowledge and a new appreciation for the needs of hospice patients.

misunderstanding or not understanding advice by doctors, and not knowing who to turn to with questions. I wanted to just let them know someone from their faith community cared and was walking with them through whatever circumstances they found themselves in.

Brother Joe and I decided to start this program with the Oratory Community, which is a small faith community where he was a member. The pastor (Father David Valtierra) was supportive of the endeavor. The provisions necessary to begin were given to us: office space, telephone, answering machine, locked filing cabinet, office supplies, and worshiping community. A health committee was formed with twelve individuals from the congregation. A health survey was distributed and from those small beginnings, this ministry took off. Brother Joe was compensated for his position as parish nurse.

I received an invitation from the associate pastor (Sister Mary Albert) of my church to speak with a group of seniors about parish nursing. This led to a presentation to the parish council and then the pastor. In my letter to the parish council, I listed what was needed to begin the program. Again, the response was enthusiastic and at that time, the president of the parish council asked me to send a letter to our pastor outlining specifics. In that letter, I asked for a modest stipend and listed the reasons why this was necessary. I felt this was a professional position, and I needed to be held accountable to the parish as a licensed professional and the parish had to recognize the position as professional. I felt a volunteer could not be held accountable or as reliable as a salaried professional in this position. If the ministry was to begin and continue, a salary needed to be entered in the yearly budget. To me, if there was no budgeted salary, there was no commitment from the parish to support or continue with the program. It had to be a covenant between both parties. I sent the letter and received a phone call from the pastor stating the parish did not feel it could support a parish nurse ministry as this time. I was extremely disappointed. The reason was financial. It would have been accepted if I had volunteered. I felt I could not accept this position without reimbursement.

After my initial disappointment, I again prayed and asked God what He would like me to do now, since I felt that the door had been closed at this point. Yet I still felt called to this ministry. I continued to work at hospice every Friday, now a full day.

I started working full time as a hospice nurse. To say that it was the best job I ever had, up to that point in time, is an understatement. This is where God was leading me, or so I thought. On April 5, 2000, my life drastically changed. I was diagnosed with breast cancer that had spread to my lymph nodes. I had a mastectomy and all lymph nodes under one arm removed. I underwent a year of chemotherapy, radiation, and more chemotherapy. My hospice "family" along with my biological family literally carried me through this difficult year.

When I was ready to officially go back to work, I did not think I could go back as a nurse out in the field. It just so happened that our volunteer coordinator was on maternity leave and I was asked to fill in for her until she came back. I agreed and was quickly oriented. I continued in this position for about six months. I was asked to coordinate the Watchman Program, which was designed to identify and train at least one individual in all congregations as a liaison between hospice and their church family. The Hospice Watchman representatives go through volunteer training and become the "hospice expert" in their church. They bring the needs of their faith communities to hospice to ensure that each person will have the opportunity to receive whatever hospice services he or she needs. The program also encourages congregation members to become hospice volunteers. I train volunteers in the hospice philosophy and every aspect of hospice so they can help educate their congregations about hospice end-of-life issues. I talk to church pastors and groups about hospice and I have met the most extraordinary people. I feel I am in the right place at the right time. Hospice Community Care funds my salary and looks at this job as a professional position and an important ministry that gives back to the community that supports us.

The "seed" that was planted sprouted many times and took many forms, but it is alive and growing. To all of those who made it possible, I offer a heartfelt thank you. To the God of creativity and compassion, who has such a sense of humor, I offer my highest praise and gratitude.

SUMMARY

In Betty's story the parish nursing narrative of nursing as ministry is told to many across multiple denominations. Virginia's developed foundational structure within a denomination through practice and written form to be passed on to many. Marie had the patience to wait and is now working in a field which will demand much in the new

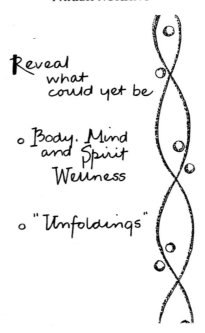

Reveal
   what
     could yet be

o Body. Mind
   and Spirit
   Wellness

o "Unfoldings"

millennium. The experience of parish nursing is different for all nurses. The 1990s produced the necessary pioneers to lay the groundwork. The soil had to be tilled, prepared, and the seeds planted for the future harvest. Different soils require different kinds of laborers to bring about the harvest of the new millennium. Parish nurses have laid the ground and are in place to contribute heavily to the wave of bioethical and resource allocation issues that lie ahead.

NOTES

1. Daniel E. Fountain, *Health, the Bible and the Church*, (Wheaton IL: The Billy Graham Center, 1989), pp. 16-29; Lloyd Kwast, "Understanding Culture," *Perspectives on the World Christian Movement*, Eds. Ralph D. Winter and Steven C. Hawthorne (Pasadena, CA: William Cary Library, 1992), p. C-3.

2. Mary Chase-Ziolek and Lawrence E. Holst, "Parish Nursing in Diverse Traditions," *Parish Nursing: Promoting Whole Person Health Within Faith Communities*, Eds. Phyllis Ann Solari-Twadell and Mary Ann McDermott (Thousand Oaks, CA: Sage, 1999), p. 196.

3. Fountain, *Health, the Bible, and the Church*, pp. 25, 27.

4. Ibid.

5. Elizabeth L. Crowell, "My Economic, Political, and Spiritual Journey to Parish Nurse Ministry. *Oates Journal* [Online] <http://www.oates.org/journal/mbr/vol-3-2000/articles/s_smith-sb3.html>. Accessed December 5, 2002.

Chapter 9

Preparation for Community-Based Work

Sybil D. Smith

Many hospital nurses in the early 1990s became weary of the "length of stay" game that maximized income margins at the sacrifice of quality patient care. Discouraged and powerless to change the system, nurses began exploring work options outside the hospital. The concept of parish nursing was emerging, and many nurses in the 1990s were drawn to explore the concept. This chapter relates the writer's assessment of the educational needs and demands of nurses who became interested in parish nursing as it unfolded in upstate South Carolina in the mid-1990s. Nonnurses were also interested in providing ministries of health and their requests for training were also considered. The continuing education programs that were developed to meet the needs of nurses transitioning from institution settings to community settings are described. Contained in this chapter are the outlines and objectives of short educational programs promoting the parish nurse journey. Not all of the nurses who explored parish nursing stayed with it. Lack of readiness for ministry was probably the biggest reason for dropping out, and several nurses strongly stated that parish nursing should be paid work. For those who discerned the call to ministries of health, hospitals often stood in the gap and provided support at a time when denominations were unresponsive.

BACKGROUND

Sister Marilyn Trowbridge pioneered the concept of parish nurse ministry across the entire state of South Carolina in the mid-1990s. Sister Marilyn's imprint was on every program that existed in the state of South Carolina in 1997. She spent over a year developing the program and began offering a ten-hour workshop in the fall of 1994.

149

At the St. Francis Hospital, in Greenville, South Carolina, Sister Marilyn gave the introductory ten-hour workshops to approximately forty nurses from seventeen parishes desiring to practice as volunteer parish nurses. In 1996, Sister Marilyn revealed to me that she would be leaving South Carolina and asked me to take her ministry. My response to Sister Marilyn was, "How can a redneck Baptist replace a Catholic nun?" Prior to this I had been an educator for the St. Francis Health System, and when I returned to graduate school I occasionally gave consultation to Sister Marilyn on program development. Sister Marilyn's response to my question was, she wanted me to take the ministry because I was Baptist. The community was 90 percent Baptist and she felt the hospital needed to be sensitive to the local culture.

A few months later Sister Marilyn left to a leadership level of service among the Franciscan Sisters of the Poor. There was a constant stream of people wanting to take the ten-hour introduction to parish nursing, which laid the initial groundwork for parish nursing. In the meantime, those who had started out with Sister Marilyn eighteen months earlier had unmet educational needs. A needs assessment from these nurses, after having practiced as parish nurses for twelve

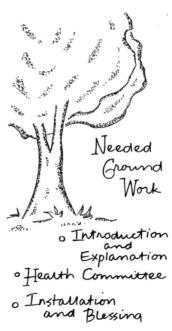

Needed Ground Work

o Introduction and Explanation
o Health Committee
o Installation and Blessing

to eighteen months, revealed a deficit in knowledge regarding family dynamics, ministry to those in the congregation experiencing brokenness, and those struggling with loss and transition issues.

Based on the assumption that brokenness in the congregation locks down the potential ministry gifts within the congregation and limits the outpouring of the benefits of the congregation to the community, I sensed an urgent need to strengthen the educational commitments to the local volunteer parish nurses in terms of the development of training modules in family dynamics and a primer for clinical pastoral education (CPE). I felt that unwrapping or unlocking the gifts in the congregation could be a lasting contribution to the poor and needful situations in the community. I felt the starting place for unlocking the gifts in the congregation was tied to identifying and unlocking the gifts within the nurses. Reflective processes, not being a part of nursing education, needed to be available for the growth of nurses in ministry. Formal CPE for nurses was not available in our area at that time.

A further assumption on my part was that the parish nurse is an appropriate member of a congregation's ministry team to the poor and needy only to the extent that the parish nurse (1) has an understanding

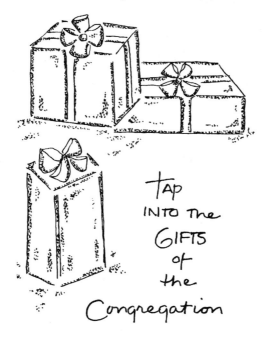

Tap INTO The GIFTS of the Congregation

of basic principles of community development, and (2) is personally on the road to spiritual maturity in grappling with the issues of justice and poverty, and realizes that caring for the poor is a biblical mandate. Community development principles are not a part of basic nursing education and have been introduced only recently into the nursing subspecialty of community health nursing. I also observed the need to develop a training module on sensitivity to cultural diversity.

St. Francis Health Ministries was the only faith-based organization in upstate South Carolina providing educational support to those in parish nurse ministries. Other organizations provided skill development for health promotion and health education, but no one was providing effective models of whole-person health that were grounded in faith and contributed to the transformation of individuals, families, and communities. Sister Marilyn was adamant that parish nursing remain ministry focused and cautioned against getting hooked in the numbers game regarding delivery of health promotion services. Ministry was believed to emerge from stewardship of one's faith after first accepting the call to become a child of God, and second, accepting the call to become a disciple of God.

Many nurses who had been employed for years in hospitals wanted to provide parish nurse ministry for their congregations. The skill set

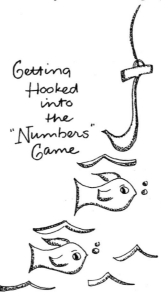

for community-based work is different than for hospital-based work. I realized that many of the knowledge deficits of those transitioning into community-based parish nursing could be met by the same training modules already identified for continuing parish nurses. A successful grant was written to the Saint Ann Foundation of Cleveland for funding the development of the training modules. Educational needs were emerging on all fronts. There were immediate needs to provide for existing parish nurses and health ministers, as well as planning for the development of the funded modules, which would be at least a year in development. In the following sections I describe how immediate needs were met, followed by a description of the funded educational modules.

IMMEDIATE EDUCATIONAL NEEDS

Provision of immediate educational resource and support for the existing volunteer parish nurses and health ministers was accomplished through local chaplains. The hospital chaplain was an approved trainer in a five-session program, "Equipping Lay People for Ministry (ELM)," developed by Dr. Ron Sunderland, Director of the Foundation for Interfaith Research and Ministry. Even though the parish nurses were professionals in the discipline of nursing, they were laity in terms of ministry. The ELM program was available to anyone in the community and became very popular. Parish nurses attended, as well as persons from congregations that did not have a parish nurse. Often, small congregations would send entire teams to the hospital to learn about visitation ministry through the ELM program. The six-week ELM program was also referred to as a program in which one could learn about story listening. A chaplain from a nearby college was recruited to develop a program specifically for educating parish nurses in bereavement ministry.

North Greenville College, a small Baptist college, was contacted about the need to develop a bereavement ministry program for laity. Dr. David Haynie, a professor at North Greenville College, developed a ten-session program that was offered in the fall and spring. Dr. Haynie was coteacher with his wife, Wanda, who was a licensed psychologist. The instructional program in bereavement ministry was available only to those active in health ministry. By the time the bereavement ministry program was in place, the hospital was offering three tiers of continuing education for parish nurses. First there was the monthly two-day introduction program that had been started by Sister Marilyn, followed by the five-session ELM program, and then the ten-week program in bereavement ministry, which focused on grief and loss issues across the life span and the appropriate intervention strategies for each age group.

Emerging from the bereavement ministry programs was the discovery of a level of spiritual woundedness among many nurses with unresolved grief and loss issues in their personal lives. Since the St. Francis Health Ministries operated from an inside-to-outside framework, I felt our commitment to support the parish nurses compelled us to be responsive to the needs of the parish nurses, believing they would not be effective in ministry with unresolved loss issues in their own lives. Dr. Haynie and his wife, Wanda, were highly regarded by the nurses, and were called on to develop an eight-week program for nurses which focused on codependency issues in relationships.

INSTRUCTIONAL MODULES FUNDED BY THE SAINT ANN FOUNDATION

Four educational modules were approved for development by the St. Ann Foundation as follows: (1) "Sensitivity to Cultural Diversity," (2) "Introduction to Community Development," (3) "Understanding God's Families," and (4) "Coping with Grief and Loss: A Pastoral Response." Each module was contracted out to an expert in the field; each instructional module was developed for the purpose of providing a resource kit for those involved in education of parish nurses and health ministers. The intended audience was nurses transitioning from years of hospital nursing into community-based work. Many of the nurses were middle-aged, near retirement, and had no desire to return to college for formal academic programs. Short continuing education programs were appropriate.

"Sensitivity to Cultural Diversity"

The module, "Sensitivity to Cultural Diversity," was authored by Dr. Karen Brown. The guiding philosophy and underlying assumptions behind the development of the module is that sensitivity to cultural diversity is a spiritual issue, dependent on one's capacity for love and ability to make space for differences.[1] The module describes the number of culturally diverse groups in the United States, discusses cultural competence, and introduces related terminology. A framework from which to assess cultural influence is presented and then applied to the three fastest-growing cultural groups in the United States.

Learning objectives for parish nurses were that they would be able to

- identify and differentiate concepts pertaining to culture, diversity, and sensitivity;
- identify and discuss the changing demographics of our nation;
- recall and describe personal experiences with diversity in culture;
- identify and discuss the concept of heritage consistency;
- identify the components of a framework (Giger and Davidhizar's Model of Transcultural Nursing) to describe and discuss cultural phenomena;
- discuss the specific cultural differences of the major cultural groups—African American, Hispanic American, and Asian American—in the United States in relation to this framework of phenomena; and
- compare and contrast health care interventions appropriate for the major cultural groups, considering the sensitivity required to achieve cultural competence.

"Introduction to Community Development"

"Introduction to Community Development," was authored by Carol Clark, MSN, RN, at Wesleyan University in Indiana. The module was developed on the assumption that health, healing, and wholeness for communities is a part of God's plan for His creation and can best be attended by the people of God who subscribe to health, healing, and wholeness for individuals, families, faith communities, and the larger environments.[2] The module presents community development concepts along with the inside/out versus outside/in frameworks. Development issues for a community are presented, along with strategies for empowering a community. The dissonance felt in community development practice is challenged. Objectives for the continuing education offering will enable participants to

- articulate foundational concepts of community development;
- identify the concepts of Christian community development;
- relate the implications of individual character with the potential for success in community development;
- distinguish between biblical and secular approaches to community, health, and medicine;
- compare and contrast transformation from within to transformation from without in a case study;
- compare and contrast the methods of practicing community development;
- summarize the process of empowering a community; and
- compare and contrast wholeness and integration among various community development approaches.

"Coping with Grief and Loss: A Pastoral Response"

"Coping with Grief and Loss: A Pastoral Response" was developed with underlying assumptions: persons are called to pastoral care ministry; pastoral care ministry is care given on behalf of the church; a pastoral care minister may be lay or professional (ordained); accepting the call to pastoral care ministry brings meaning and purpose to one's life; ministry opportunities exist in the crises of life; and as a pastoral care minister one is reconciled to self, others, and God as one suffers and matures through the onslaughts of life becoming a wounded healer. The course introduces students to the manner in which society at large and individuals in particular understand and cope with dying, death, and the grief process following a loved one's death. The program was designed for an eight-week format.

Objectives for the module are as follows:

- Identify the historical routes that have led to the present state of grief awareness and grief education
- Appreciate the breadth of human responses to grief as these may be discerned from literature and psychological research
- Describe the process of normal grief
- Identify the tasks of mourning
- Identify barriers to effective grief work
- Apply listening skills to care of bereaved people
- Identify factors that contribute to complicated grief

- Identify indications that a bereaved person is stalled in the process of mourning
- Identify issues integral to children's mourning needs
- Describe the place of grief education in preparing children to cope with bereavement
- Relate the importance of adult modeling of mourning to children's grief education
- Contrast dying as a special (particular) situation in living, and death as the outcome of dying, not its equivalent
- Describe palliative care for the dying
- Identify the role of hospice
- Relate the contribution of funeral practices to the mourning process
- Describe the social rituals and values of funeral practices
- Identify and explore personal attitudes and hesitancies regarding funeral practices
- Identify culturally determined factors related to death and dying
- Recognize that attendance to cultural factors will likely determine the degree to which an individual is able to cope with grief and loss
- Identify religious factors which shape attitudes and practices
- Identify life losses and changes other than death that evoke experiences of grief
- Identify the degrees to which losses other than death may exacerbate grief over deaths of loved ones

The "Coping with Grief and Loss: A Pastoral Response" module was authored by Dr. Ron Sunderland of Houston.[3] Dr. Sunderland's ELM five-week program of study was so well received, he was contracted to develop this module as a follow-up to ELM. Also it was felt that the continuity of a stream of lay ministry education would build the foundation for care team ministries in the future.

"Understanding God's Families"

"Understanding God's Families" ended up being three four-hour workshops. The guiding philosophy and assumptions include the idea that persons are born or adopted into families of origin and that families of origin are centers from which hearts and minds are formed.[4] The three workshops are titled, Sanctity of the Family, Family Resiliency, and Family Dynamics. They are presented from a family systems perspective with a focus on what is required to endure the onslaughts of life as individuals and families. Virginia Wepfer, MSN, RN, C, who holds a master's specialty in family health, authored the materials.

The Sanctity of the Family module compares and contrasts American cultural values, family values, and Christian values as they relate to sacredness of the family. Sacredness of the family is further related to family development and family structure.

In the Family Resiliency module, resiliency is defined in terms of the relationship between family stress and coping and family adjustment and family adaptation. The impact of family stressors on the internal and external environments of individuals is explored in terms of problem solving, appraisal, and worldview. Factors that contribute to family resiliency are explicated and related to family nursing distinguishing between family-focused care and family-centered care.

The Family Dynamics module details family systems, communication patterns, and family functioning. Attachment bonds are explored across the family developmental stages. Interaction patterns, power alliances, and changes in divorce and remarriage are compared and contrasted.

Two hundred sets of the modules were initially run and advertised in the quarterly health ministries newsletter that had a distribution of 2,000. Most were purchased from outside the state. At the local level, we had the largest response when the "Sensitivity to Cultural Diversity" programs were taught.

THE REALITIES

There was some criticism from the academic community, which felt that nurses gravitating to community-based work would benefit from completing a BSN rather than becoming involved in continuing education. I do support that a BSN is minimal preparation for community-based work, but most of our attendees were nurses close to retirement or not even nurses at all. The background of all activities was filled with the noisy rhetoric of the International Parish Nurse Resource Center, the Health Ministries Association, and local hospitals competing for market share even with their community-outreach programs such as parish nursing and ministries of health.

In addition to managing the immediate educational needs and the development of the funded modules, there was a need to offer short programs related to spiritual formation, prayer, pain, and suffering. This need was unexpected and carried me into a deeper level of study and prayer for preparation. These programs were offered multiple times a month, were well attended, and are outlined in the appendixes to this chapter. They were promoted on a local religious television station, which boosted attendance to waiting-list levels because I found it easier to work with groups of ten to fifteen at a time. We had over 300 attendees the last five months I was involved with the program. The St. Francis Foundation, which funded my salary, was pleased with the community response, and provided adequately for my clerical and resource support to manage the operation. The foundation also encouraged and provided for times of personal renewal and retreat. On occasion I was asked to recruit some of the volunteer parish nurses to provide community services on behalf of the hospital. This did not go over well. The nurses were volunteers to their respective congregations and felt no obligation to be a hospital volunteer, despite the hospital's heavy investiture in their educational development. I worked with two congregations in underprivileged neighborhoods and was able to recruit volunteers for a few specialty events in those locations.

I was the only doctoral-prepared parish nurse coordinator in upstate South Carolina; my calling was clear and specific for educational and resource support for ministry formation; and I was given space by the St. Francis Foundation to live out that calling. It was difficult for me to serve as a parish nurse in my own congregation because my church was in a different county from my employer, which meant my personal community of faith was marketed by a competing health system. Eyebrows were raised in my community of faith because I was employed by a Catholic facility and involved in church-related activities among multiple denominations. In my own congregation I volunteered my parish nurse services in nonintrusive ways, and in underprivileged churches as needed around the county at first; but later my calendar was filled with teaching the short programs on prayer, healing, pain, and suffering. Monthly network meetings also had to be coordinated. These were opportunities for the parish nurses to come together for fellowship and updates on health promotion activities. The St. Francis Foundation also provided two-day retreats in the fall and spring for parish nurses, bringing in national conference leaders. The retreats were coordinated through my office and held at nearby facilities.

Of the thirty people who completed the three-tier program of health ministry education, the two-day introduction, the five-week ELM or story listening program, and the ten-week bereavement ministry program, only three are not in some type of ministry of health today. One went on to complete a counseling degree, and another completed a quarter of CPE. Many of those who attended only the two-day introductory program are no longer involved in ministries of health. I listened to stories of nurses who were disappointed when their congregations showed no interest in ministries of health.

REFLECTIONS AND SUMMARY

My personal study and growth during the parish nurse journey carried me to a new level of service and stewardship of my faith. There came a point in the development of the education and resource support for parish nurses that an appropriate and practical level of continuing education was established. I had groomed a nurse educator, who had gone through all of the programs and had completed a unit of CPE years earlier, to take over the ministry. Administratively the decision was made not to honor my recommendation for replacement.

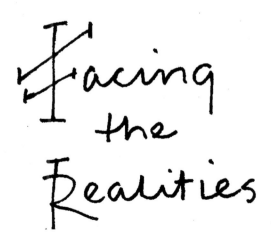

Facing the Realities

The vacancy stood for six months and a nurse without education experience was placed in the role.

Today I continue with the same vision and calling and am involved in education and resource development for ministries of health at the academic level. I use the same mission/ministry framework in the development of programs to impact systems of care, affirming the values of sanctity and dignity at end of life. Some of the short programs I developed for parish nurses on health, healing, prayer, pain, and suffering served as springboards to three-hour, full semester credit college courses.

This chapter has summarized the history of a parish nurse ministry of a particular hospital and at the same time presented educational resources that can stimulate new programs of parish nurse ministry. The foci of the programs of education are rooted in a level of religious calling where one finds meaning and purpose as he or she becomes a steward of the faith.

APPENDIX A:
HEALTH, HEALING, AND WHOLENESS SERIES

Overview

The concepts of health, healing, wholeness, prayer, and suffering are explored from a biblical worldview and presented in a series of four workshops for adults. A youth version has been developed for eight one-hour sessions taken from Workshops One through Three.

Objectives

Workshop One

- Assess various definitions of health and relate them to premodern, modern, and postmodern medicine.
- Describe various concepts of healing and relate them to behavior-driven versus culture-driven healing strategies.
- Compare and contrast secular versus biblical views of healing.
- Discuss the process of wholeness.
- Relate health and healing to wholeness and the driving force of love.

Workshop Two

- Formulate a definition of spirituality.
- Identify and assess some of the spiritual issues of life.
- Relate the spiritual issues of life to Christian development.
- Differentiate among types of prayer.
- Relate prayer and the journey to wholeness.

Workshop Three

- Define suffering; describe various types of suffering; and relate pain and suffering.
- Relate the experience of suffering to beliefs about suffering and opening the discourse on spirituality.
- Describe ways to alleviate suffering and the process of inviting reflections on suffering.

Workshop Four

- Compare and contrast various approaches to nursing and health ministries in congregations.
- Describe components of a mission-ministry approach to nursing and health ministries.
- Differentiate between parish nursing and health ministries.
- Clarify values and priorities of your congregation.
- Formulate a start-up plan for a congregational health program.

APPENDIX B:
YOUTH PROGRAM—PRAYING FOR HEALTH,
HEALING, AND WHOLENESS

Overview

The concepts of health, healing, wholeness, prayer, and suffering are explored from a biblical worldview and presented in an eight-session format with worksheets provided for each session.

Copyright: Sybil D. Smith, PhD, RN.

Purpose

To answer these questions:
- Why pray?
- To whom do we pray?
- For what do we pray?

Objectives

Session One

- Identify multiple reasons we are drawn to prayer.
- Describe six types of suffering.
- Compare and contrast two parts of suffering.

Session Two

- Define health and terms related to health.
- Describe six types of illness and their underlying issues.
- Relate underlying issues to health problems.

Session Three

- Define healing and terms related to healing.
- Compare and contrast secular versus biblical views of healing.

Session Four

- Describe the process of wholeness.
- Relate wholeness to faith formation.
- Compare and contrast brokenness and wholeness.

Session Five

- Relate suffering to prayer for health, healing, and wholeness.
- Describe techniques of suffering.

Session Six

- Describe the biblical view of God.
- Describe the biblical view of the person.
- Discuss the need for the Triune God of Relationship.

Session Seven

- Compare and contrast five types of prayer.
- Discuss praying for wholeness.

Session Eight

- Discuss the journey from brokenness to wholeness.
- Relate spiritual issues to behavior options.
- Relate spiritual issues and the journey to wholeness.

NOTES

1. Karen M. Brown, "Sensitivity to Cultural Diversity: An Instructional Module" (Greenville, SC: St. Francis Health Ministries, 1998). Funded by Grant 9/3-SAF-44, Saint Ann Foundation, Cleveland, OH.

2. Carol Clark, "Introduction to Community Development: An Instructional Module" (Greenville, SC: St. Francis Health Ministries, 1998). Funded by Grant 9/3-SAF-44, Saint Ann Foundation, Cleveland, OH.

3. Ron Sunderland, "Coping with Grief and Loss: A Pastoral Response," (Greenville, SC: St. Francis Health Ministries, 1998). Funded by Grant 9/3-SAF-44, Saint Ann Foundation, Cleveland, OH.

4. Virginia C. Wepfer, "Understanding God's Families" (Greenville, SC: St. Francis Health Ministries, 1998). Funded by Grant 9/3-SAF-44, Saint Ann Foundation, Cleveland, OH.

Chapter 10

Program Evaluation

Susan Fuentes

Evaluation is sometimes regarded as a dirty word, especially in faith communities where we regard results and success to be up to God. It is true that we will never know the full results or outcomes of our work. However, it is necessary to have a sense of responsibility for the stewardship of time, money, and of resources and of being accountable for our actions. In order to know if we are on track, we must pause to evaluate these actions. Only then can corrections be made and effectiveness increased.

Evaluation is defined as the systematic collection, analysis, and reporting of information for decision making. It includes various methods such as interviews, focus groups, observation, videotaping, questionnaires, tests, and statistics.[1] This chapter reviews the salient reasons for doing evaluation and some of the evaluation methods used by parish nursing programs.

REASONS TO EVALUATE

Quality Improvement

The most important reason to evaluate the activities of your program is to learn more about what is being done correctly so it can be duplicated, and to recognize where improvements are needed. Failures cannot be turned into successes unless the problems are identified and corrected. In order to improve the quality of the services provided there must be a process to systematically review past actions and produced outcomes. This is an important facet of community development, as well as an expected standard of parish nursing practice. The standards clearly state, "the parish nurse initiates and partici-

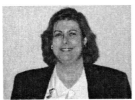

Susan Fuentes, MSN, RN, is Vice President and Director of the QueensCare Health and Faith Partnership (QHFP) in Los Angeles, one of the most successful parish nursing programs in the country. QHFP is an organization-based parish nursing program involving over sixty congregations, nonpublic schools, and community agencies, with an annual budget of over $1.4 million and a paid staff of twenty-three registered nurses and nine support staff. They provide lifesaving health screening, health counseling, health education, case management, and spiritual care to the low-income and uninsured in metro Los Angeles. QHFP is part of the QueensCare health system that includes five community clinics, ancillary services, a specialty panel, and six contracted hospitals.

Susan earned her master's degree in nursing at Azusa Pacific University in 1997 along with clinical nurse specialist certification and completed her thesis on "The Effects of Parish Nursing on Client Wellness." She is involved in her local congregation by serving as a care minister, a member of the Ministry Council's Community Outreach Division, and on the Lake Avenue Foundation Board of Directors. She also serves on a statewide steering committee for compassionate end-of-life care, the California Coalition for Compassionate Care. Susan has received numerous awards for her work with underserved communities, most notably the Alumnus of the Year Award from Point Loma Nazarene University and induction into Azusa Pacific University's Academic Hall of Fame in 2000.

pates in self-evaluation and evaluation of the overall health ministry program in order to acknowledge nursing actions and improve the quality of services provided."[2] Evaluation is key as responsible stewards accountable for our work.

Celebration

Unless we can review our actions we cannot celebrate them. Many programs are so busy doing activities that there is little time to stop, reflect, and celebrate the accomplishments. Celebrating revitalizes workers involved in the program and also stimulates outsider interests. No one wants to get involved with a program that is unsuccessful; it is important to demonstrate and build on your successes.

Reporting

Every program is accountable to some higher authority, whether governing board's members, the community served, or outside investors. Reporting is important in conveying program accomplishments, budgetary concerns, and population served. Reporting should be done on a regular basis—preferably monthly, quarterly, and annually.

Reports must be relevant and easy to understand. You must determine what information needs to be reported, systematically collect the data, and then report it in concise but simple terms. For instance, most people prefer graphs and illustrations to tables of numbers. Include examples and success stories that illustrate what the numbers mean. It is much more interesting to hear a report about a health fair if specific stories or results are discussed. Compare the impact of the second example given in Box 10.1 to the first example. Which one stirs your emotions and calls you to act? Do not be afraid to tell the human side of the story, such as, "Two of the forty-six women who attended the cervical cancer screening had never been screened before,

---

BOX 10.1. Reporting

Ineffective Reporting

On October 16, the Health and Faith Collaborative sponsored a Health Fair.

Effective Reporting:

On October 16, the Mytown Health and Faith Collaborative sponsored a Health Fair. Twenty local agencies participated in the Health Fair, including the Mytown Hospital, the Public Health Department, Sam's drugstore, the Mytown school district, and sixteen local churches. The Health Fair was attended by 285 people. Ninety percent of those attending live in Mytown, and 60 percent were parents of children age five or younger. Forty-six children were immunized at the Health Fair, 150 people were screened for high blood pressure, and 200 nutrition packets were given away. Those who attended were highly satisfied with what the fair had to offer, and most said they hoped that Mytown would hold the fair next year.

Source: Adapted from *We Did It Ourselves: An Evaluation Guidebook,* SRI International, 2000.

and one of them was referred for suspicious findings." This demon-strates to even the most medically unsavvy person the importance of holding such screenings in safe and trusted environments such as faith communities.

Communication

Communicating your results and learning experiences is another excellent reason to evaluate. If you do not have a clear understanding of program accomplishments, how can you share them with others? Evaluation data will communicate the specific benefits the program offers constituents and the wider community. This is crucial if parish nursing programs are to validate their relevance and influence on the health care of their community. Part of this communication may take the form of brochures, pamphlets, annual reports, and articles for the media and professional journals.

Dissemination

Often forgotten is the necessity, even duty, to disseminate evalua-tion findings. Many outside communities are eager to learn about the success of your program so they may replicate it. Parish nursing is on the cutting edge of a wider national movement to bring health and faith together, and to form collaborations in order to do so. It is cru-cial to the future of parish nursing for us to document our knowledge and experiences, and thus contribute to the learning of others.

EVALUATION METHODS

Participant Evaluations

The most common way of evaluating program activities is to have participants fill out a short survey. The survey should reflect the kind of service provided, whether an educational class, a health screening, or a one-on-one consultation with a parish nurse. The survey should be in the native language of the participant, written for the appropri-ate educational level, and take no longer than five minutes to com-plete. When writing survey questions stop to think what you want to know. It sounds simple, but many questionnaires have unnecessary questions. If you are not going to report on a certain topic, do not collect information on it.

Surveys or questionnaires should have at least one question that measures the participant's satisfaction with the program provided. For sample questions see Box 10.2. Keep in mind when designing the survey that it will need to be tabulated. Open-ended questions are important in learning what participants thought of the program, but are difficult and time consuming to tabulate. Questions that use true/false or yes/no answers are easier to tabulate but do not give a lot of extra information. Rating scales are easy to tabulate and give a bit more information than the yes/no method, but sometimes participants struggle with choosing a number. Always leave space for participants to give specific feedback. Even if you choose to not publish the responses, they provide essential feedback and give participant's permission to verbalize what is important to them.

Health Committee Reports/Program Surveys

In parish nursing programs it is important to remember that the individual participant is not the only client of the program. Evaluation must also include the health committee and the organizational leadership. In faith communities this is the pastor, priest, rabbi, or other spiritual leader. The questions should reflect on the usefulness of the parish nursing program, and the parish nurse specifically. This evaluation not only yields good information about how the faith community feels about the program, but also gives insight into the community's understanding of and involvement in the program. Thus, it becomes a teaching tool to facilitate better communication and fuller understanding (see Figure 10.1).

BOX 10.2. Sample Client Survey Questions

1. What service did you receive today?
2. Do you feel your needs were met? Explain.
3. What did you like about the program?
4. What changes would you suggest for the future?
5. Would you recommend this program to your friends and family? Why?
6. Additional Comments:

FIGURE 10.1. Parish Nurse Program Evaluation

Faith Community: _____

Parish Nurse: _____

Evaluator: _____ Date: _____

1. What is your opinion of the program?

    ❑ Excellent, is invaluable and must be continued

    ❑ Good, continue program

    ❑ Satisfactory, continue program but needs improvement

    ❑ Unsatisfactory, program ineffective, discontinue

2. Describe overall interactions with the program leadership.

    ❑ Effective   ❑ Ineffective

3. If the answer is ineffective, please state the reason why, and how we can improve. _____

    _____

    _____

4. In what ways has the program been helpful to your faith community? _____

    _____

    _____

5. Please suggest ways we could further benefit your ministry. _____

    _____

    _____

6. Other comments and suggestions: _____

    _____

    _____

    _____

Please take a moment to evaluate the effectiveness of your parish nurse. If you would like these comments kept confidential, please let us know.

Rating Scale: 3 = Excellent, 2 = Satisfactory, 1 = Needs Improvement

PARISH NURSE ROLES	RATING	COMMENTS
Health Educator—Promotes an understanding of the relationship between body, mind, and spirit by providing health education classes and other activities that address the assessed needs.		
Health Counselor—Is on site four to eight hours per week to provide individual health consultations. Makes home, hospital, church, school, and phone visits as requested. Responds to health concerns of clients promptly and professionally. Provides crisis intervention as needed.		
Volunteer Coordinator—Facilitates the use of volunteers in your health ministry. Helps develop and coordinate a health committee; works with them to plan, implement, and evaluate effective health programs.		
Health Screening/Referral—Provides appropriate health screenings, and refers clients to appropriate health care when needs are beyond nurse's abilities. Facilitates utilization of congregational/community resources by staff and constituents.		
Case Manager/Advocate—Assists persons to understand and navigate the health care system. Acts on clients' behalf to ensure they are treated justly. Provides follow-up to make sure persons are receiving needed care.		
Pastoral Caregiver—Serves as part of the ministry team. Assists clergy in providing prayer, healing services, sacraments, etc. as requested. Provides spiritual care to individuals and families.		
Other—Maintains confidentiality at all times. Meets with leadership regularly, and keeps site leadership informed of activities. Maintains open communication between health committee, site leadership, and program leadership. Operates within the values and beliefs of your faith.		

The health committee should also have ongoing evaluations. Every health committee meeting should have a time to reflect on the previous month's health event. This can be done informally with each member sharing his or her feedback, or formally, with participation numbers, issues addressed, and referrals reported. Participant surveys may be tabulated and included in this evaluation. The key to this evaluation is learning from mistakes and planning for the future. Whatever method is used, results should be documented and plans set for the future (see Figure 10.2).

Parish Nurse Self-Evaluation

The parish nurse has a responsibility to set outcomes and evaluate responses for individual clients and for the programs provided. The parish nursing standards of practice require self-evaluation as part of professional development.[4] One way to incorporate this into a systematic approach to evaluation is to include parish nurse self-evaluation as part of the annual performance review. This ensures a collaborative process to the evaluation of parish nurse performance (see Chapter 11). This self-evaluation could also be part of a mentoring relationship with feedback, support, and accountability being given by the mentor. Self-evaluation must be an honest exercise in order to pinpoint strengths and weaknesses. Although it is much easier for the parish nurse to provide yes/no answers or rate herself or himself on a scale, requiring the nurse to respond narratively will cause deeper reflection and elicit more meaningful data. It is important to follow up on these revelations with any necessary resources or support. Some sample questions are listed in Box 10.3.

Statistical Data

It is important for most programs to collect and report statistical data on services provided, to whom, and how much. We count the number of blood pressure exams, how many were abnormal, and how many people were referred. By gathering the numbers we can predict and detect information about the design of the program, and generate information for decisions about why things are happening. Anyone

FIGURE 10.2. Health Cabinet Program Evaluation Tool

FAITH COMMUNITY: _____

EVENT/PROGRAM: _____

DATE/TIME: _____

1. Who took a leadership role? _____

2. What were the goals of this event? _____
   _____

3. Did we accomplish the goals set? If not, why? _____
   _____

4. Total participants: _____

5. What age group(s)? _____

6. Strengths/successes: _____
   _____

7. Lessons learned: _____
   _____

8. Plans for improvement: _____
   _____

9. Comments: _____
   _____
   _____

Health Cabinet Chair: _____

who has been in program management knows that numbers are necessary for demonstrating the effectiveness of your program. Fortunately, this method of evaluation is fairly straightforward. It can be as simple as paper forms or as technical as computer spreadsheets and databases.

BOX 10.3. Parish Nurse Self-Evaluation Questions

❑ How well do you manage your time?
❑ What are your specific strengths that make this kind of nursing a good match for you?
❑ In what areas do you feel least qualified to do your job?
❑ Describe how you carry out each of the parish nurse roles.
❑ List three goals for yourself to achieve in the next year and how you plan to achieve them.
❑ What can be done by the program leadership to help you?
❑ If you were in charge for the day and could change anything about our program, what would that be?

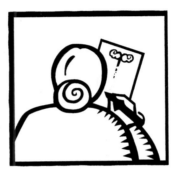

Regardless of the method, the important thing is to figure out what kinds of information you need. It is quite frustrating to collect information, tabulate and report it, only to find out you missed a very important measurement. Equally as frustrating is to collect information that you cannot or will not ever use. Therefore, think carefully about what kinds of information you need before designing your measurement tool. Some important data to include are age, gender, type of insurance, date of service, type of visit (telephone, home, hospital, office), new or established client, services received (blood pressure, spiritual support, crisis intervention, case management, etc.), and referrals given. Anything you want or need to know about your client population should be on your measurement tool. It may be helpful to involve the parish nurse(s) in designing the tool itself. Remember, the easier it is for the parish nurse to collect the data, the better the data you receive will be.

Outcome Measurement

One reason faith communities may not be eager to evaluate is that typical evaluation methods do not capture the benefits and transformation they see. Unlike process evaluation, measuring outcomes ask a different set of questions—what effect did the program have on the recipient? Thus, outcome evaluation measures transformations versus transactions. It does not measure what we have done, but what impact we have had on the recipient. It also serves a quality improvement function as it allows us to evaluate the program's contributions and to improve on service delivery and productivity.

Outcome engineering (OE) is one form of outcome measurement that is being utilized by many parish nursing programs across the United States.[5] It is an Internet-based system that uses program recipient stories to quantify program contributions. OE provides a method for evaluating the results of traditionally hard-to-measure activities and services such as complex, multistrategy work with individuals and their environments. It offers a common, outcome-based language for discussing program performance and a set of standard scoring algorithms for gauging success relative to earlier periods or in comparison to other programs tackling similar outcome challenges. Cumulative scores are computed as a program takes actions that lead to development/transformation for the clients and other key stakeholders and reports these gains.[6]

Outcome engineering has several key concepts that set it apart from other methods. First, it does not take undue credit for client transformation, but measures the program's contributions to a client's transformation. Many aspects are out of the program's control. Thus, we are contributors to improving the health outcomes of our clients, but not producers. Second, it is a people-focused measurement tool. Expected outcomes are defined in terms of the program's effects on the people it serves, such as "teenagers who make health choices," or "people who promote health in their communities." Third, it requires that outcomes are subjective. Numbers and other objective measures tend to narrow and quantify the broader reality of human science into something it is not. Real-life struggles and transformations cannot be objectified. Fourth, it builds capacity by bringing other key stakeholders into the planning, implementation, and evaluation process. It gives "extra credit" to programs that link with other providers and make use of volunteers. This is significant, since parish nursing does not just simply solve problems or meet needs in isolation, but builds a network of collaborators.

Whether using outcome engineering or another outcome measurement tool, there is no getting away from the need to demonstrate program effectiveness. It is no longer enough to demonstrate the amounts and types of services a program provides. Programs must be able to provide proof of the effectiveness and success of their interventions.

By developing an evaluation strategy that uses a variety of methods, is ongoing, and is systematic, the parish nurse program will have the necessary data to document its effectiveness and benefits and to improve the quality of services. As parish nursing is a complex role and depends on many other factors, using one or two evaluations tools will not provide sufficient information or evidence. The evaluation data must communicate the full and rich story of transformation that occurs with clients.

NOTES

1. SRI International, *We Did It Ourselves: An Evaluation Guide Book* (Sacramento, CA: Sierra Health Foundation, 2000).

2. Health Ministries Association, Inc., and American Nurses Association, *Scope and Standards of Parish Nursing Practice* (Washington, DC: American Nurses Publishing, 1998), p. 15.

3. Fuentes, Susan (2002). "QueensCare Health and Faith Partnership Program Evaluation," unpublished document. QueensCare, 1300 N. Vermont Avenue, Suite 907, Los Angeles, CA, 90027; <www.QueensCare.org>; 800-454-1800.

4. Ibid., p. 16.

5. Barry M. Kibel, Pacific Institute for Research and Evaluation, <www.pire.org/resultsmapping/>.

6. Barry M. Kibel (1999). "Why Outcome Engineering?" unpublished paper. Results Mapping Laboratory, Pacific Institute for Research and Evaluation, 104 S. Estes Drive, Suite 206, Chapel Hill, NC 27514; 919-967-8998; <www.outcome engineering.com>.

Chapter 11
Developing Resources

Susan Fuentes

Parish nursing practice is a uniquely reciprocal design in which the parish nurse must interrelate to other health ministers, health care providers, and community resources in order to bring optimum health to the client system—whether individual, family, faith community, or neighborhood. Some resources are quite obvious, such as people and money. Others are not as straightforward but are just as important, such as building a strong community coalition and drawing on the resources of the community. This chapter addresses developing resources from an organization-based paid parish nursing model. However, whether paid or volunteer, congregation or organization based, the key concepts remain the same.

HUMAN RESOURCES

Hiring

The most important resource for a successful parish nursing program is the parish nurse. Her or his unique experience, education, skills, and gifts are imperative. A parish nurse is "a registered professional nurse who serves as a member of the ministry staff of a faith community to promote health as wholeness of the faith community, its family and individual members, and the community it serves through the independent practice of nursing."[1]

Parish nursing is a specialty practice that requires a unique set of skills, experience, and education.

Finding the right person for the job is not easy. Creative recruiting and interviewing strategies must be used to find the most qualified candidate. Simply putting an advertisement in the local newspaper will not yield good results. Try using denominational periodicals and meetings, health career fairs, job postings at churches and schools of nursing, and word of mouth.

Before interviewing potential candidates, a job description must be developed. Without a job description it will be difficult to determine if a candidate is right for the position, and the correct approach for relevant interview questions. When looking for suitable candidates to interview, narrow the search by having applicants complete an interest form with questions about the person's faith background and current faith commitment. In order to function within the faith-community setting and perform the expected duties and responsibilities, the nurse's faith commitment is most relevant. Do not be shy when asking about an applicant's level of faith about commitment. It is not the particular religion or its practices that are important, but the vitality of the person's spiritual journey.

Parish nurses are required by the nature of their work within faith communities to have a strong faith commitment.
- Do you participate in a particular faith tradition?
- In what ways do you participate in the life and ministry of your church/temple/synagogue/mosque?

Other important factors include the applicant's ability to communicate effectively, previous parish nursing or community health experience (a BSN with public health nursing experience is recommended), flexibility, a team player mentality, ability to function independently, possession of an automobile and insurance, and willingness to work varied hours including weekends. Professional liability insurance will be needed to cover the parish nurse's practice, and can be purchased by the sponsoring organization, the faith community, or the parish nurse.

Orientation/Training

The orientation period is an extremely important tool for the faith community and parish nurse to build the foundation for learning and working together. Expectations must be clarified and a team must be built. Orientation to a new role is very stressful, with many new things to learn and process, but it is also very rewarding. It is important that the orientation and training be both didactic and experiential. There are many great resources for the new parish nurse to consult. However, as important as books, videos, Web sites, etc. are, nothing can replace the actual hands-on experience.

Parish Nurse Web Resources

www.ipnrc.parishnurses.org

www.healthministriesassociation.org

www.QueensCare.org/healthandfaith.html

www.tdh.state.tx.us/library/nursing.htm

www.chausa.org/parish/nursing.asp

http://groups.yahoo.com/group/ParishNurse/

www.cord.edu/dept/parishnursing/

www.carroll.edu/parishnurse/index.html

The full orientation should last four to six weeks, including on-site training with a preceptor. This important hands-on training allows the orientee to practice what has been learned didactically. The best orientation program combines the parish nurse's strengths, experience, and interests with additional resources to increase competency in the multifaceted parish nursing role. To do this, one must assess current competency and then design an orientation strategy for each individual. It is helpful to have the parish nurse take an active part in the assessment and design. The orientation program should include the following:

- history and philosophy of health ministry/parish nursing
- organizational mission, governance, policies and procedures
- job description and scope of practice
- spirituality and health/spiritual care
- communication and assessment skills
- community health promotion
- working with the health committee/volunteers
- cultural diversity
- community resources/tour of the community
- health program planning, implementation, and evaluation

- participatory health/empowerment
- accountability—documentation and reporting

Orientation should not be considered successfully concluded until the parish nurse has completed a competency checklist. The checklist should include skills and knowledge needed for basic performance based on the job description, such as health assessment, performance of screening procedures, safety procedures, infection control, documentation, use of office equipment, etc.

Development/Mentoring

Parish nurses are health care generalists in that they need to know a little about a lot of things. They are responsible for the whole spectrum of human development and disease, from cradle to grave, from physical to spiritual health. It is not possible for a parish nurse to know it all. It is critical that she or he knows where and when to find help, has supportive backup, and accepts her or his limitations. Strategies to help development include professional education and inservices on timely and relevant topics, spiritual reflection and support, fellowship, retreat and renewal, and the mentoring relationship.

Mentoring comes from the tradition of apprenticeship: working alongside another more experienced and skilled craftsman to learn a trade. It also includes the dimension of friend or advocate which is important in building confidence and independence in addition to skill. These are of utmost importance to parish nurse development due to the independent nature of the role. Developing the skills and knowledge base of the parish nurse is important, but nurturing the unique personhood and spiritual being is even more important. One does not need to be a parish nurse to be a good mentor. Clergy, other health professionals, retired persons, and basically anyone who has the time and interest in the personal and spiritual development of the parish nurse is qualified.

Discipline

Included in any type of employee relationship, whether volunteer or paid, are performance review, counseling when performance is below standard, and termination if necessary. Discipline should always be corrective and positive, with the goal of improving performance and confidence. Ongoing communication with the parish nurse is essential and should include both positive and corrective feedback. There should be no surprises when conducting the annual review.

Written documentation of both overperformance and underperformance is important. Written documentation can include employee commendation memos, disciplinary memos, feedback from others closely involved with the program, and finally, first, second, and final warnings of termination. Corrective action should always include specific examples and should strike a balance between compassion and truth. Finally, if the parish nurse is unable or unwilling to correct performance, and the goals of the program are not being met, it is in the best interest of all to terminate the relationship.

FINANCES

It is well known that any successful program in ministry cannot last long without adequate finances. How does one find resources to start and keep a parish nursing program growing? There are four primary ways to garner financial support. The successful program will use a variety of resources, not depending on one or another. The most important thing to do before looking for outside funds is to articulate the vision, mission, and goals of your program. This demonstration of need for your services will be a critical step in garnering financial resources.

Grants/Public Funding/Contracts

Many organizations, especially faith communities, are wary of seeking funding from outside sources. There are many different kinds of funders, both private and public, that have legitimate interests in the health of communities. As long as mission, philosophy, and goals can be aligned, these funds are great resources for parish nursing programs. The key is, what are the expectations of the grantee? Can the grantee be faithful to the grant requirements? Many faith communities do not wish to be answerable to any outside organization, especially the government. However, it is important to note that faith communities are already accountable to many, including their governing board, members, and ultimately to God. As long as goals are congruent, there should be no problem being accountable to yet another. It is when programs promise to do things they cannot deliver, or the financial backer does not have a full understanding of the unique mission and goals of the faith community, that problems erupt.

Private foundations, in particular, are great sources of funds for development of parish nursing programs. They usually have broader guidelines for what they will fund and less stringent reporting requirements. There are many great resources for learning about foundations nationwide that list current requests for proposals (RFPs). Look on the Internet and for grantsmanship centers or seminars in your area. The most important thing to remember when seeking funding is that the grantor is dependent on the grantee to accomplish its funding goals. If you feel you have a good program that answers a need in your community, do not be afraid to sell your unique ability to put the funder's money to good use.

Other sources of funds are public grants and contracts. These are called "carve outs" or "block grants" and are for specific projects such as teen pregnancy prevention, tobacco cessation, health services for the uninsured, or access to rural health care. They usually have very complex applications and stringent reporting requirements. Public funding is a very real option if your program can identify a specific service rendered or education program provided and you have access to a grant writer.

Currently, the government has committed to eliminating barriers that faith groups experience when applying for federal funding. There is a strong movement to recognize faith communities as legitimate providers of health and social services. This is an important step in recognizing the contributions of parish nursing programs, but we must exercise caution as we explore and enter these new relationships.

Fund-Raisers and In-Kind Giving

These important areas of financing for parish nursing programs are often overlooked. One of the unique strengths of faith communities is the ability to supply in-kind support and to do their own fund-raising. In-kind support can be members donating needed items to the parish nurse program, staffing the program with volunteers, and providing unreimbursed use of the facility, utilities, office equipment, and supplies. Fund-raisers can be very successful methods of raising money, and they have the added benefit of bringing people together and generating fun. Bake sales, dinner dances, auctions, raffles, and special offerings can be valuable assets. They also provide a more ongoing funding source than other methods.

Private Donations

Developing a donor base of private individuals can be very profitable. This can be an elaborate series of strategies such as monthly plea letters, annual events such as golf tournaments and auctions, or potential donor parties. It can also be as simple as putting donation envelopes in a newsletter or brochure. It is important to communicate to private donors how their money will be used—the more specific the better. Developing gift levels or special funding projects can be helpful to donors who want to fund something very specific such as immunizations for uninsured children. Using success stories and thank-you letters from participants is heartwarming and also very effective. The fact is, individuals give organizations over 75 percent of their financial support, so do not overlook this valuable resource.[2]

Third-Party Payment

Perhaps the most important, but least understood, funding resource for the ongoing development of parish nursing programs is the ability to collect reimbursement for services from third-party payers. These include insurance companies, federal, state, and county public assistance programs, and co-payments by participants. Although organization-based programs have the advantage here, congregation-based programs that have adequate technological and human resources can be just as effective at collecting payment.

In order to collect reimbursement, parish nursing programs must first set up a fee schedule for services rendered. The most successful method of doing this is to follow already established reimbursement codes and fees. Medicare and Medicaid have set fee schedules and procedure codes that cover many of the services parish nurses provide.[3] A set of unique procedure codes and fees for those services not already covered can be created using customary charges.

Using these codes and fees, along with an accounting of monthly activities provided, one can report the dollar cost and value of said services and potentially bill for them. If parish nursing is to exist in the current health care environment, such accounting will be needed to demonstrate validity and cost-effectiveness of services provided. An example of this is the QueensCare Health and Faith Partnership, which was able to account for over $2 million of free health care it provided to its community in 2000-2001 (see Figure 11.1).[4]

FIGURE 11.1. QueensCare Health and Faith Partnership Encounter Form[5]

Last Name:		First Name:		MI:	DOB:

Account #:	Address:		Zip Code:

Insurance Plan:	Language Code:	Ethnicity Code:	Gender:

Type of Visits:

499390 Office Visit	499372 Telephone, Intermediate
499232 Hospital Visit	499373 Telephone, Complex
499348 Home Visit	499280 Health Promoter Visit
499354 Clinic Visit	499380 New Client
499371 Telephone, Brief	499400 Screening Visit

Referrals Made:

499271 QueensCare	499275 Church/Program Staff
499272 Other Clinic	499276 Social Services
499274 PMD	499278 Hospital

Services Provided:

499401 Health Education, 15 mins	490712 Oral Polio
499402 Health Education, 30 mins	490718 Tetanus
499403 Health Education, 45 mins	490732 Pneumococcal
499404 Health Education, 60 mins	490744 Hep B
499078 Health Education, Illness	490730 Hep A
499360 Case Management, 15 mins	499450 Health Appraisal
499361 Case Management, 30 mins	486580 Tuberculosis, PPD
499362 Case Management, 60 mins	47325 Men's Cancer Scrng
499363 Transportation Assistance	48155 Women's Cancer Scrng
499241 Disease Mngmnt, 15 mins	42090 Scoliosis Screening
499242 Disease Mngmnt, 30 mins	42499 Vision Screening
499262 Spiritual Support	42551 Hearing Screening
499273 Crisis Intervention	43350 Lice Screening
499279 First Aid	43658 Blood Pressure Scrng
490648 Hib Vaccine	41025 Pregnancy Test
490657 Influenza Vaccine	42962 Diabetes Scrng, Glucometer
490701 DPT	44829 Cholesterol Screening
490707 MMR	499414 Height/Weight Screening

Other Activities:

499411 Health Education, Group—30 mins	499374 Health Records Review
499412 Health Education, Group—60 mins	499416 CPR Class
499413 Parenting Classes	

Location Code:	Provider Code:	Date of Service:	Signature:

COMMUNITY DEVELOPMENT

Parish nursing and health ministry are based on the community development principles of relocation, reconciliation, redistribution, holistic approach, grassroots, church-based authority, developing community leadership and assets, and empowerment.[6] Whether referring to the faith community or wider community these principles apply—a parish nurse without community support and resources is like a fish out of water. A parish nursing program cannot function effectively without community influence and support. Without community involvement, the parish nurse would be isolated from the very needs and resources necessary to do her or his work.

The first thing to remember when serving the community is to become the learner and observer before setting goals and implementing plans. The community is not simply an important partner, but the primary driver of the health ministry vehicle. There are three primary steps to becoming a mutual partner within the community: (1) networking with the community, (2) assessing both community assets and needs, and (3) building on the strengths of the community and establishing collaborative relationships.

Networking

There is no better way to become acquainted with community and allow them to become acquainted with you than to network. Networking should be a two-way street. That is, join every group that has to do with community health, with the primary objectives to learn and observe, but also bring information and resources to these groups. In addition to attending meetings, walking the streets of the community, eating at the local hangouts, and taking rapid transit are also effective strategies. Bringing your own personal and professional expertise and gifts to these encounters is important to building a relationship of mutual trust and respect. As you spend significant time with community members, they will get to know you and see that you care about them. The kinds of resources you bring to a community are unique and important, such as connections with other health professionals, knowledge of how to access health care providers, experience with many health issues, and the ability to make connections with health-related organizations. Do not forget to recognize, however, that the community has many resources beneficial to your work. They are your allies in meeting the needs of the community.

Community Assessment

Many programs, especially in health care, see the community either as a cacophony of need or as a marketplace for selling their product. Both of these views are flawed and will not bring health and wholeness to a community. The community must be appreciated for its unique and diverse strengths. Only then can one realize what the community brings to the equation, what the program has to offer, and how the program and the community can work together. By pooling their resources they can do much more than either one alone.

There are different assessment methods, each with pros and cons. Interviewing key informants paints the broadest strokes, but it is cumbersome and time intensive to analyze and summarize the data. Observation is important and useful, but can take a lot of time and is difficult to document. Administering surveys is a common form of assessment and easy to document and tabulate, but falls short in its ability to capture a complete and true picture of the community (see Figure 11.2). It is important to know the right questions to ask, as well as how and when to ask them. For example, a four-page form handed out as people leave the worship service at lunchtime is not going to yield much helpful data; and sometimes people tell you what they think you want to hear even with the best designed questionnaire.

Capacity Building/Collaboration

Identifying with a community's capacity to bring positive changes in lifestyle or health-seeking behavior is probably the most rewarding part of the parish nurse role. Collaboration, or working toward a common good with uncommon partners, is a lot of work and can at times seem unproductive. It is akin to the ripple effect on a pond. For days, weeks, months, and even years you keep throwing little pebbles into the water producing nothing but a small, ineffectual ripple. Eventually, the pebbles pile up and suddenly the water begins to be redirected. The trick is to keep everyone working on the same project—or pile of pebbles—at the same time.

FIGURE 11.2. Health Ministry Survey[7]

The health committee of _____ is planning health programs for our church/agency and those served by our outreach programs. You can help by completing this confidential questionnaire. This information will be tabulated and used for program development.

1. Male ❑ Female ❑
2. Age: 0-12 ❑ 13-19 ❑   20-40 ❑   41-65 ❑   65+ ❑
3. Primary language spoken_____
4. Do you live: Alone ❑   With Family ❑   Apartment ❑ House ❑
5. Do you have someone you can rely on when you need help? YES ❑ NO ❑
   What is your relationship to that person?
   Family ❑ Friend ❑ Work Associate ❑ Church Associate ❑ Other _____
6. Employment status: Part-time ❑ Full-time ❑ Unemployed ❑ Retired ❑
7. Are you covered by an insurance plan? YES ❑ NO ❑
8. Health conditions in your family (please check all that apply)

   ❑ Asthma   ❑ High Blood Pressure
   ❑ Arthritis   ❑ Lung Disease
   ❑ Cancer   ❑ Mental Illness
   ❑ Depression   ❑ Substance Abuse
   ❑ Diabetes   ❑ Tuberculosis
   ❑ HIV   ❑ Weight Problem
   ❑ Heart Disease   ❑ Other _____

9. Which of the following would you use if they were offered at this church/ agency?

   ❑ Blood Pressure Screening
   ❑ Cholesterol Testing
   ❑ Blood Sugar Testing
   ❑ Stop Smoking Classes
   ❑ Nutrition or Healthy Cooking
   ❑ Help with an Addiction
   ❑ Weight Control Program
   ❑ Parenting Classes
   ❑ Exercise or Aerobics Classes
   ❑ Other _____

CAPACITY BUILDING IS . . .

the development of an organization's core skills and capabilities, such as leadership, management, finance and fundraising, programs and evaluation, in order to build the organization's effectiveness and sustainability. It is the process of assisting an individual or group to identify and address issues and gain the insights, knowledge, and experience needed to solve problems and implement change. Capacity building is facilitated through the provision of technical support activities; such as coaching, training, site-specific technical assistance, problem solving, and resource networking.[8]

The most important thing to remember in building collaborations is that everyone has something to bring to the project, and may have different reasons for participating. The trick is to figure out the various motivations and to bring them in alignment. If all can agree on a common goal and participate equally to make it happen, the project will be successful. In addition, it is important to note it is not always the final product that brings the best learning and success. Sometimes it is in the act of working together that transformation happens. For example, if the common goal is to clean up the trash and graffiti in the neighborhood, but in the process of doing so the group develops into an effective and energized team, not only will the neighborhood be cleaner and less dangerous but there will be a stronger sense of cohesion and vision that can drive the group to future successes. If one or two people do it by themselves, they will simply have a cleaner neighborhood for a few days.

Thus, building collaborations and capacity is building a team (see Table 11.1). Every person on the team has something unique to bring to the work, and a specific reason for participating. The parish nurse is not necessarily the leader of the team and, in fact, should not be the leader. Leaders need to come from within the community in order for the team to be long term and self-sustaining. You know you have been successful at collaboration and capacity building when your absence from an important meeting goes unnoticed.

In parish nursing the key community leader and collaborative institution is the health committee (see Box 11.1). This committee consists of people who have caught the vision of better health and wholeness for their community and are invested in making it happen. They

TABLE 11.1. Team Characteristics

What Helps a Team to Be Effective?	
Effective Team	**Ineffective Team**
Personal needs and team objectives integrated	Mistrust, fear
Diversity of ideas encouraged; collaboration among team members	Members withdrawn and passive
	Play-it-safe attitude
Goals clearly defined, understood, and accepted	Conflict suppressed, smoothed over, denied, avoided
Members interdependent	Overabundance of harmony—often superficial
Initiative and coordination often shared by members	Ideas that falter due to lack of support, examination, and/or understanding
Acceptance of team members for who they are	Many hidden feelings
Resources among members identified and used effectively	Members wanting others to assume responsibility
Genuine respect among members	Counterdependence
Open, clear, two-way communication	Occasional fights over leadership
Decisions made by consensus	Desire to be shown and told exactly how to do things
Influence based on ability and expertise	Team does not own the goals
High trust and cohesiveness	Rigid conformity of behavior
Equal and valued participation by all team members	Influence based on position
	Emphasis on individual performance
	Team maintenance ignored

may be health professionals, but it is not necessary. Sometimes the most effective health cabinet member is the church secretary who knows everyone, or the retired teacher who has extra time to invest. Every person on the committee should have a responsibility, whether chairperson, secretary, publicity, refreshment coordinator, treasurer, etc. The committee must meet at least monthly to plan and implement health classes or events and to sustain momentum. The committee, not the parish nurse, should be responsible for program outreach, implementation, and evaluation. The parish nurse brings clinical expertise and health resources to the team. The more decision-making authority this committee has, the more successful the programs will be.

In conclusion, anyone can set up shop at a church, temple, or mosque, supply a parish nurse, a blood pressure cuff and stethoscope, and have a parish nurse program. To be a transforming change agent in people's lives takes much, much more. It takes time, energy, and the

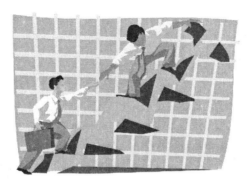

BOX 11.1. Steps to Becoming a Successful Health Committee

1. Establish a foundation of trust.
2. Define clear roles and responsibilities.
3. Allow sufficient planning and start-up time.
4. Create specific and measurable goals and objectives.
5. Acquire sufficient resources and support to meet the goals and objectives.
6. Implement an effective needs assessment for creative problem solving.
7. Conduct meaningful monitoring and evaluation.

know-how to find and develop many kinds of resources. The parish nursing program without a full complement of resources is like a beautiful fruit tree on a deserted island. The tree may yield delicious and nourishing fruit, but with no way to harvest it, both tree and fruit will wither and die. Likewise, a parish nurse program that exists in isolation, without tapping into the resources and needs around it, will be ineffective. With its community fully involved and leading the way, the program will nourish and bless those it serves.

NOTES

1. Health Ministries Association and American Parish Nurses Association, *Scope and Standards of Parish Nursing Practice* (Washington, DC: American Parish Nurses Publishing, 1998).

2. AAFRC Trust for Philanthropy/Giving USA, 2001.

3. Practice Management Information Corporation, *International Classification of Diseases and Clinical Modification,* Los Angeles, 2001. <www.medicalbookstore.com>.

4. QueensCare Health and Faith Partnership Annual Report, June 2001.

5. Fuentes, Susan (2002). "QueensCare Health and Faith Partnership Program Evaluation," unpublished document. QueensCare, 1300 N. Vermont Avenue, Suite 907, Los Angeles, CA, 90027, <www.QueensCare.org>, 800-454-1800.

6. Wayne Gordon, Speech at 13th Annual Christian Community Development Conference, Dallas, Texas, November 29, 2001.

7. Fuentes (2002).

8. California Wellness Foundation (2001). "Reflections on Capacity Building," 2(2), p. 4. Report in a series published by The California Wellness Foundation, 6320 Canoga Avenue, Suite 1700, Woodland Hills, CA, 91367, <www.tcwf.org>.

PART IV:
PARISH NURSING
AND END-OF-LIFE ISSUES

Chapter 12

End-of-Life Issues

Karen M. Brown

Literature supports a general disappointment that people have experienced concerning care at the end of life. Nurses are present when patients and families are confronted with health crises, and decisions concerning end-of-life issues are focal. In advocating for the patient and family, nurses must communicate and coordinate holistic care, care of the mind, body, and spirit, at the end of life. How will parish nurses become involved in end-of-life issues? The creation of a transitional bridge between life and death considers the spiritual and religious aspects of nursing care. Parish nurses of the future, as an integral part of communities of faith, will be confronted with end-of-life issues as congregations become more involved in ministries to the aging.

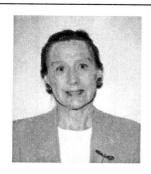

Karen M. Brown, DSN, APRN, BC, began a thirty-five-year career in nursing with a BSN from Alverno College in Milwaukee, Wisconsin. Experiences include military nursing, staff nursing, home health, parish nursing, and education. She has been employed as faculty at Baptist College of Charleston, University of South Carolina at Spartanburg, and Clemson University teaching primarily child health and community health nursing. She holds an MSN in community health from Clemson University and a doctorate of science in nursing in health care policy from the University of Alabama at Birmingham, and she obtained certification from ANCC as specialist in community health. Presently Karen is employed as a health advocate, consultant, and educator in the business sector.

DYING IN THE UNITED STATES

Death is the greatest certainty of life and presents many challenges to the individual, family, health care provider, clergy, and community. Life on earth is the time we experience between conception and death, a time that the discipline of nursing has supported with dignity and compassion. All people on earth are terminal for a variety of reasons, some people just sooner than other people. Since the 1950s, medical advancements to prolong life have forced individuals, families, and health care providers to make decisions about when and how a life should end. The decision-making process for end-of-life care involves patient rights, family rights, state's rights, and the responsibility of the federal government.

David Kessler, friend and protégé of Elisabeth Kübler-Ross, also discusses the rights of the dying.[1] He utilizes reflections from his personal experiences and insights to teach others how to work with the dying and how to listen. Seventeen principles are offered by Kessler to help the individual, family, and friends learn to face death with compassionate dignity. Communication is stressed for the dying family member as well as participation of family members to express emotions and choices as they face death together. In discussions with Mother Teresa, Kessler learned that death is "a going home to God."

Prior to the 1940s, death was a family affair in which the family cared for the dying and prepared for the funeral with the help of their children, church, and community. The hospital gradually became the transition place for death beginning in the 1950s and 1960s, and soon the dying individual was removed from family and community to reside in a sterile intensive care unit. This created a hospital experience in which loved ones were unable to be part of the dying process. Lack of knowledge, fear, and misunderstandings began to cloud decision making and communication during these times. This has gradually been changing with the hospice movement in the 1980s and the palliative care movement of the 1990s.

Hospice is a philosophy of caring for loved ones while avoiding aggressive medical care and promoting a more natural death by providing comfort care and pain management. Hospice, however, is usually recommended only when the physician determines that nothing will help prolong life or change physically, and the person will die within six months. Admission criteria to hospices typically require, for insurance reimbursement purposes, a diagnosis of terminal illness with less than six months to live. Palliative care focuses on quality of life rather than length of life, and the holistic caring of patients that are not responsive to curative treatment; it does not contain a time element. Many health care providers and communities are not familiar with the relatively new concept of palliative care; the political arena for reimbursement is even more complicated for palliative care than for hospice.

The tremendous advances in medical technology have prolonged life but have not defined the quality of the extended life, nor has holistic care (care of the mind, body, and spirit) for the individual and family been accomplished. This is highlighted by the U.S. Supreme Court decision in 1997, which considered the constitutional right to physician-assisted suicide. The court rejected all claims to a constitutional right to support physician-assisted suicide.[2]

DESCRIPTION OF END-OF-LIFE ISSUES

Numerous phenomena are embraced as individuals are confronted with the term *end-of-life issues.* An end-of-life continuum of care is described by the American Nurses Association (ANA) and begins with comfort care and the alleviation of pain and suffering. This progresses to the self-determination act, and choices concerning hydration and nutrition, do-not-resuscitate decisions, and the possible request for assisted suicide and active euthanasia. Because these issues are value laden and politically charged, the American Nurses Association has published position statements to support and provide appropriate holistic care at the end of life.[3]

Presently, of the two million people who die each year in America, 80 percent die in hospitals, hospices, or nursing homes, and two-thirds of these are from chronic disease such as cancer or heart disease.[4] The circumstances are not important. The patient could be a neonate, the eldest member of our society, a young accident victim, or a person at midlife with a debilitating illness. All have a right to informed decision making and to exercise personal choices related to the quality of life at the end of life. All have a right to comfort and closure in this life and preparation for what they believe comes after death.

A survey by George H. Gallup International Institute to investigate the role of spiritual beliefs in preparing for, and dealing with, death found that for a person to find comfort in dying, human contact is important.[5] This was described as sharing fears, having someone there, and touching and holding someone's hand. The survey found that spiritual comfort was also important to the participants, and was described as prayer or becoming spiritually at peace. Spiritual comfort was looked for primarily from family (81 percent) and friends (61 percent), rather than clergy (36 percent), doctors (30 percent), or nurses (21 percent). Participants also had a strong preference to die at home (70 percent) rather than in the hospital (17 percent). Concerns at the end of life were expressed as being vegetable-like (73 percent); not saying good-bye (73 percent); great physical pain (67 percent); care of family or loved ones when gone (65 percent); and death being cause of stress for loved ones (64 percent). Only 28 percent of the survey participants prepared living wills or advance medical directives and only 10 to 12 percent of those informed their health care providers that they had a living will. The opportunity for education and communication related to spiritual and end-of-life issues by nursing for the individual and family is present.

Informed decision making of the individual safeguards the medical, nursing, and health care professions by obtaining consent and protecting the autonomy or the right of the individual to make his or her own decision. This process should occur over time and includes the input, assimilation, and decision phases based on the information presented and the worldview of the individual in light of his or her values and beliefs.[6] Health care providers assume that the adult, competent patient should make his or her own decisions. The multicultural climate of the United States presents a challenge to the hospital policies in the treatment of the terminally ill and dying. Cultural differences affect ethical decision making. Some cultures do not value individualism as much as Western societies do. The linguistic, educational, and emotional barriers to effective communication can also alter the decision-making process.

Professional nurses have a responsibility to society, and the American Nurses Association is a working member of the Consortium for Quality End-of-Life Care. This is a multidisciplinary organization which focuses on the challenges of end-of-life care and the current inadequacies of the health care system, that is, pain management and physician-assisted suicide, which need to be addressed by federal and state governments.[7] Immediate actions that can be taken by nursing organizations are presented in Box 12.1.

HISTORICAL PERSPECTIVE

The historical perspective on the end-of-life concept began with the founding of the Euthanasia Society of America in 1938. Euthanasia literally means a "good death" and has been taken to mean the "act

---

BOX 12.1. Actions That Can Be Taken by Nursing Organizations

1. Disseminate the Consortium recommendations to board of directors, leadership members, and other constituencies through newsletters, electronic communications, journals, etc.
2. Endorse the Last Acts' *Precepts of Palliative Care*.
3. Include End-of-Life Care in each organization's strategic planning process.
4. Include articles related to End-of-Life Care in each organization's journal.
5. Include End-of-Life Care content in all national, regional, and local meetings.
6. Highlight national and regional activities, research, and educational opportunities related to End-of-Life Care in organizational communication mechanisms such as Web site, newsletters, electronic communications, etc.
7. Identify member expertise in End-of-Life Care.
8. Adopt or endorse existing position statements on End-of-Life Care.
9. Review existing standards, guidelines, and position statements regarding End-of-Life Care.
10. Catalog organizational resources related to End-of-Life Care.
11. Establish organizational mechanisms to monitor End-of-Life Care activities.
12. Collaborate with other organizations to advance the agenda for End-of-Life Care.
13. Disseminate End-of-Life Care information to local and national media.
14. Disseminate existing knowledge of pain and symptom assessment and management to members.
15. Include End-of-Life Care in the organization's research agenda.

Source: "Designing an Agenda for the Nursing Profession on End-of-Life Care," Workshop Funded by the Open Society Institute and Project on Death in America (PDIA). Report Released November 1999 by AACN, <www.aacn.org>, accessed November 22, 2002. Used with permission.

of putting to death someone suffering from a painful and prolonged illness or injury."[8] The ANA position is not open to the possibility of participation in assisted suicide due to its covenant to respect and protect human life. Euthanasia can be active, the hastening of death by someone's actions, or passive, the hastening of death by not acting. It can be further divided into voluntary, involuntary, or nonvoluntary depending upon whether the patient consents, does not consent, or cannot consent to the action or situation. The present social struggles with the continuum challenge nurses and other professionals to improve end-of-life care so that assisted suicide will not be possible.

The social, ethical, and legal controversies of end of life were observed in 1975 with the Quinlan case in New Jersey. The Quinlan family undertook a prolonged legal battle and the state court granted the family permission to remove life support.[9] In 1976, the California Natural Death Act was passed by the California legislature and represented the first state to address end-of-life issue. In 1990, the federal government became involved in end-of-life decision-making issues when the Cruzan case was heard by the U.S. Supreme Court.

The Patient Self-Determination Act of 1990 (PSDA) was passed by all federal legislators and is utilized in fifty states and the District of Columbia. The overall purpose is to inform and educate people about their rights to direct holistic health care and encourage them to communicate these choices to their health care provider. The law provides the requirement for information but does not indicate how it should be executed.[10] The readability of many of the states' advance directives have been found to be difficult for the majority of the population.[11] Discussion with individuals and families is necessary for clarification.

In 1998, the Florida Commission on Aging with Dignity developed a more readable document that is an acceptable legal document for end-of-life choices in thirty-three states.[12] The document is titled "Five Wishes" and answers five pertinent questions that inform the doctor, family, and friends of how the individual wishes to be treated if seriously ill and unable to make certain decisions. These questions are about (1) the person I want to make care decisions for me when I can't, (2) the kind of medical treatment I want or don't want, (3) how comfortable I want to be, (4) how I want people to treat me, and (5) what I want my loved ones to know. This document helps to exercise the le-

gal and moral rights to decide medical care if seriously ill and antici-
pating death.

Another important consideration for the decision-making process
in end-of-life care is directly related to the financial climate of the situation. Death and financial pressures are positively correlated. One-
third of all families coping with a terminal illness will add poverty to
their list of concerns. Ten percent of the health care dollar goes to the
terminally ill. Money is also becoming a decision-making factor in
end-of-life care. Within the current social discussions "a right to die
may become a duty to die" as economic pressures escalate and the
terminally ill exist in an atmosphere in which they are not valued.[13]
Caplan, as cited in Bilchik, noted that managed care's economic in-
centives have turned "end-of-life issues upside down."[14] In the past,
people advocated for a living will because doctors were paid to perform and people were afraid they would do too much, especially unnecessary procedures. Presently, the fear of getting too little care in
regard to managed care is growing. The uninsured in the current system of health care are silent when it comes to support for the legaliza-
tion of assisted suicide.

THE SPIRITUAL DIMENSION

The spiritual dimension of life integrates values and beliefs, and is
fundamental to the way one thinks, acts, and feels in health, illness, at
the end of life, and in the transition to death. The close relationship of
spirituality to religion is seen in its everyday usage as found in
Merriam-Webster's Collegiate Dictionary.[15] The first three mean-
ings of spirituality refer to ecclesiastical law, the church, or sensitivity to religious values. Julia Emblem found the terms *spirituality* and
religion to be interchangeable in literature.[16] After further study, religion was determined to be "a system of organized beliefs and worship which the person practices" and spiritual was "a personal life
principle which animates transcendent quality of a relationship with
God or god being." It was concluded that religion was subsumed in
the broader concept of the spiritual.

Florence Nightingale's manuscript, *Suggestions for Thought,* discussed her philosophy and introduced her spiritual beliefs as a sense
of a "presence higher than human, the divine intelligence that creates,

sustains, and organizes the universe, and an awareness of our inner connection with this higher reality."[17] Travelbee was one of the first nurse theorists to acknowledge the spiritual dimension by emphasizing the importance of finding meaning as a process in understanding health.[18] Other theories of nursing that contribute to the concept of spirituality are those of Neuman, Newman, Watson, and Parse. They place spirituality as a major focus such that the removal of the concept will create a significant shift in their theory.[19] Nursing is involved in the spiritual dimension of caring for the dying. Parish nurses are in the unique role of creating a transitional bridge of holistic caring for the dying.

Kessler wrote about the comfort and peace that is found in spirituality at the end of life.[20] At the closing of life people realize they must let go and have faith. Most are familiar with the steps described by Kübler-Ross in facing death: denial, anger, bargaining, depression, and acceptance.[21] Kessler has suggested the five steps to spiritual reconciliation: expression, responsibility, forgiveness, acceptance, and gratitude. Healing takes place as anger is expressed, responsibility is accepted for choices, forgiveness is extended to oneself and others to make us whole, and acceptance of death allows all life to be complete, no matter how short. The spiritual journey creates a feeling of gratitude for life, both the good times and the bad. In a national survey by the George H. Gallup International Institute, "the overarching message that emerges is that the American people want to reclaim and reassert the spiritual dimension in dying."[22]

SUMMARY

This chapter discussed dying in the United States and provided an overview of end-of-life issues. The historical perspective on end-of-life issues was presented along with consideration of the spiritual dimension. The role for professional nurses in end-of-life issues is obvious, and a foundation has been laid by the ANA for nurses to become active participants, walking alongside individuals and families at end of life. Parish nurses can expand the role of professional nursing within the church community and encompass the needs of parishioners, contributing to a peaceful death for congregation members as well as outreach to the community. The experience of nonhospice hospital nurses with patients encountering end-of-life choices is different from community-based nurses because hospital nurses do not have long-term relationships with patients and their families.

If scholars ponder the complexity of end-of-life issues, think how much more difficult it is for patients and families, especially if they have defaulted to "at need" decision making. Because nurses interact with vulnerable patients and families at end of life, nurses need to be educationally prepared and spiritually reconciled to their own dying. Since spirituality encompasses what one believes about living and dying, the nurse's view of spirituality impacts her or his capacity for intervention strategies at end of life.

NOTES

1. David Kessler, *The Rights of the Dying: A Companion for Life's Final Moments* (New York: Harper Collins, 1999).

2. American Nurses Association, *ANA Praises Supreme Court Decision on Physician-Assisted Suicide* (Washington, DC: Author, 1997, June 26).

3. American Nurses Association, *Position Statement: Promotion of Comfort and Relief of Pain in Dying Patients* (Washington, DC: Author, 1991, September 5); American Nurses Association, *Position Statement: Nursing and the Self-Determination Act* (Washington, DC: Author, 1991, November 18); American Nurses Association, *Position Statement: Forgoing Artificial Nutrition and Hydration* (Washington, DC: Author, 1992, April 2); American Nurses Association, *Position Statement: Nursing Care and Do-Not-Resuscitate Decisions* (Washington, DC: Author, 1992, April 2); American Nurses Association, *Position Statement: The Non-Negotiable Nature of the ANA Code for Nurses with Interpretive Statements* (Washington, DC: Author, 1994, December 8); American Nurses Association, *Position Statement: Assisted Suicide* (Washington, DC: Author, 1994, December); American Nurses Association, *Position Statement: Active Euthanasia* (Washington, DC: Author, 1994, December 8).

4. Choice in Dying, *Facts About End of Life Care* (New York: Author, 1996, March).

5. George H. Gallup International Institute, *Spiritual Beliefs and the Dying Process* (Princeton, NJ: Author, 1997), pp. 7-12.

6. Linda L. Barret, "Supporting End of Life Decision Making," *Activities, Adaptation and Aging*, 1994, 18(3/4): 77-88.

7. American Nurses Association, "ANA Focuses Efforts on Improving End-of-Life Care," *The American Nurse*, 1997, May/June, 10.

8. American Nurses Association, *Position Statement: The Non-Negotiable Nature*.

9. Choice in Dying, *Facts About End of Life Care*.

10. Case Management Advisor, "Help Patients Make Informed Decisions About the End of Life," *American Health Consultants*, 1996, 7(3): 29-32.

11. Barbara B. Ott and Thomas L. Hardie, "Readability of Advance Directive Documents," *Image: Journal of Nursing Scholarship,* 1997, 29(1): 53-57.

12. Charles A. Corr, Clyde M. Nabe, and Donna M. Corr, *Death and Dying, Life and Living* (Belmont, CA: Wadsworth, 2000), pp. 434-435.

13. Gloria S. Bilchik, "Dollars and Death: Money Changes Everything, Now It's Entering the Debate Over the Right to Die—with Explosive Results," *Hospitals and Health Networks,* 70; 1996: 18-22.

14. Ibid., p. 21.

15. Frederick C. Mish, Editor in Chief, *Merriam-Webster's Collegiate Dictionary,* Tenth Edition (Springfield, MA: Merriam-Webster, 1993).

16. Julia D. Emblem, "Religion and Spirituality Defined According to Current Use in Nursing Literature," *Journal of Professional Nursing,* 1992, 8(1): 41-47.

17. Janet Macrae, "Nightingale's Spiritual Philosophy and Its Significance for Modern Nursing," *IMAGE: Journal of Nursing Scholarship,* 1995, 27(1): 8-10.

18. Joyce Travelbee, *Interpersonal Aspects of Nursing,* Second Edition (Philadelphia, PA: FA Davis, 1971).

19. D. S. Martsolf and J. R. Mickley, "The Concept of Spirituality in Nursing Theories: Differing World-Views and Extent of Focus," *Journal of Advanced Nursing* 7; 1998: 294-303.

20. David Kessler, *The Rights of the Dying.*

21. Elisabeth Kübler-Ross, *On Death and Dying* (New York: Macmillan, 1969).

22. George H. Gallup International Institute, *Spiritual Beliefs and the Dying Process,* p. 1.

Chapter 13

A Role for Parish Nursing
in End-of-Life Care

Janet Timms

The health industry is moving toward ambulatory- and community-based care in multiple settings and there is an increased awareness and obligation to support quality of life and peaceful death at the end of life. Some of the factors that have necessitated increased attention by the nursing profession to the provision of care at the end of life include (1) the demands of the aging population, (2) the social demand for improved end-of-life (EOL) care which has been expressed to some degree by attempts at national legislation on assisted suicide and euthanasia, (3) a burdened health care system, and (4) prevalence of diseases such as cancer, AIDS, and other chronic diseases.

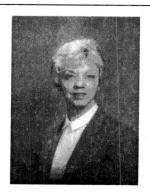

Dr. Janet Timms is Associate Director and Associate Professor in the School of Nursing at Clemson University, Clemson, South Carolina. She received baccalaureate and master's degrees in nursing from Clemson University and a doctorate in education from the University of Georgia. She is a gerontological clinical nurse specialist with teaching, research, and administrative responsibilities in graduate and undergraduate education. Her research interests in gerontology focus on end-of-life care, caregivers of the elderly, and gerontological nursing education.

DEMANDS OF THE AGING POPULATION

Currently, individuals aged sixty-five and older comprise approximately 13 percent of the population. During the period 1989 to 2030, the aged sixty-five-plus population is predicted to double and is expected to account for 22 percent of the population in the year 2030.[1] In the beginning of the twentieth century, most Americans did not live past age sixty-five, but life expectancy has increased dramatically since 1900, and today approximately three-fourths of all deaths are at ages sixty-five or older.[2] These demographic changes caused by the graying of the baby boom generation require increased emphasis on the importance of end-of-life care for health care providers.[3]

SOCIAL DEMAND FOR END-OF-LIFE CARE

Concerns about the need for increased attention to end-of-life care are exacerbated by the inadequate number of nurses providing care and by inadequate preparation in end-of-life care. The nation is experiencing an acute nursing shortage that is predicted to become worse over the next ten to fifteen years. *Critical for Care: The South Carolina Nursing Workforce, 2001 and Beyond,* reported by Loquist and Pease, cited multiple contributing factors to the current and predicted shortage.[4] Factors contributing to the nursing shortage include

1. a large cohort of nurses reaching retirement age who are expected to leave the profession in record numbers by 2010,
2. a marked shortage of nurses with baccalaureate and higher degrees to practice in an increasingly complex health care delivery system,
3. a shortage of qualified nurse faculty, limiting the ability to increase enrollment in nursing programs,
4. a declining interest among young women choosing nursing as a career,
5. growth in the aging of the general population with chronic diseases increasing the demand for nursing services, and
6. work environment issues that negatively impact recruitment and retention.

The problem of the inadequate number of nurses providing care for patients and the inadequate number of faculty providing instruction is compounded by the inadequate knowledge of end-of-life issues. It is well documented in the literature that nurses, faculty, and other health care professionals have inadequate academic preparation related to end-of-life care.[5] With these issues confronting both providers and recipients of care, it seems increasingly clear that all nurses must assume personal responsibility to acquire the necessary preparation to provide the care that is needed now and in the future. They must assure that the scope and standards of practice of their nursing specialty will enable them to meet patients' health care needs.

THE BURDENED HEALTH CARE SYSTEM

Projections of national health expenditures indicate an approximate doubling of health spending from $1.1 trillion in 1997 to $2.2 trillion by the year 2008. Health care expenditures, as a share of the gross domestic product (GDP), are predicted to rise from 13.5 percent in 1997 to 16.2 percent by 2008. Expenditures on health care include the cost of physicians' services, hospitalizations, home health care, nursing home care, medications, and any other goods and services used in the treatment or prevention of disease.[6] Despite the projected acceleration in health spending, growth is expected to remain well below the long-term historical average spending, due to effects of managed care, the rising uninsured population, and a projected slower growth in Medicare spending.[7] Overall, public funding, including federal, state, and local programs, pays for approximately 45 percent of the nation's personal health care costs and 72 percent of Medicare beneficiaries' health costs.[8] Although managed care plans may reduce or help control national health expenditures, the personal and financial impact of the cumulative effect of chronic illness, impairments, and disability is a major concern among the growing population of the elderly and their caregivers. Health care can be a major expense for older Americans, especially for individuals with limited incomes. Although average dollar expenditures on health care increase with income, the relative burden of health care costs is much higher among lower income households and households in the middle of the income distribution.[9]

Societal needs are driven by both the needs of patients and the needs of health care agencies for nursing expertise in managing care for the increasing number of elderly discharged with shortened length of stay in acute care settings to home and community settings for recuperative care. Diminishing resources and increasing need have historically characterized the elderly population, which frequently exhibit multiple chronic illnesses, limited resources, and limited health care access. Nurses functioning in a variety of community-based organizations provide an ideal solution to the provision of care and leadership needed to assure that health care requirements of this vulnerable and culturally diverse population are met.

PREVALENCE OF DISEASES

Six disease groups account for almost two-thirds of all personal health care expenditures. When expenditures are analyzed by diagnosis, diseases of the circulatory system (i.e., heart disease, stroke, and hypertension) are most costly, followed by diseases of the digestive system (including all dental expenditures). The remaining most costly disease categories, in descending order, are mental disrders, injuries and poisoning, nervous system and sense organ diseases, and respiratory diseases.[10]

Aging has long been associated with an increased prevalence of chronic disease and death, and poor health behaviors are leading contributors to morbidity and premature mortality. Research evidence indicates that behavior change, even in later life, is beneficial and can result in improved disease control and enhanced quality of life.[11] Improved disease control may translate to reduced spending for long-term care. While most spending for long-term care in the United States is for nursing home and other institutional care, the majority of older persons with disabilities are not institutionalized but reside in the community and receive assistance from informal and unpaid caregivers. As these individuals age and reach the time when end-of-life care is needed, the health care system will have an inadequate supply of nurses prepared to provide symptom management, palliative, and end-of-life care. As the aging population increases the demand for long-term care in the community, important questions will be raised about who will provide the care and how it will be financed.[12] Can our overburdened health system afford only referrals from parish nurses when confronted with these issues? Parish nurses are in a unique position to respond to these challenges and opportunities and it behooves this group of professionals to examine the *Scope and Standards of Parish Nursing Practice* (1998) to determine whether their patients' needs may be more effectively met with some modification of current parish nursing standards.[13]

The rationale for suggesting that nursing organizations examine their current standards is based on the recent organizational support from several important nursing, medical, and state initiatives which have addressed concerns about some of the current deficiencies in end-of-life care. Examples follow:

1. The International Council of Nurses issued a mandate in 1997 stating that nurses have a unique and primary responsibility ensuring that individuals at the end-of-life experience a peaceful death.[14]

2. In recognition of the universal need for humane end-of-life (EOL) care, the American Association of Colleges of Nursing (AACN), supported by Robert Wood Johnson Foundation, convened a roundtable of experts in 1997 to stimulate discussion and initiate change on end-of-life care. The AACN roundtable's ethicists and palliative care experts developed "Fifteen Competencies Necessary for Nurses to Provide High Quality Care to Patients and Families During the Transition at the End-of-Life." These competencies from the AACN Peaceful Death Document are intended to affect what is taught in nursing schools to increase the focus on symptom management and psychosocial support.[15]

3. Representatives from twenty-three organizations, organized by AACN, met in June 1999 at George Mason University in Fairfax, Virginia, to draft an agenda for the nursing profession to improve end-of-life care. The meeting resulted in a list of priorities for improving end-of-life care. The meeting was organized by AACN (with grants from Soros Foundation, Open Society Institute, and Project on Death in America). Priorities established by the group were

   - developing nationally recognized nursing standards for the care of the dying,
   - improving end-of-life care content in undergraduate and graduate education,

- increasing nursing research on end-of-life care,
- increasing nursing efforts to remove regulation reimbursement barriers to comprehensive palliative care services,
- improving mechanisms for sharing information on end-of-life care between nursing organizations and individual nurses, and
- making the relief of pain a priority in improved end-of-life care.[16]

4. The Joint Committee of Accreditation on Health Care Organizations now mandates good end-of-life care within inpatient settings.[17]

5. Americans for Better Care of the Dying (ABCD) has a draft list of legislative goals for Congress to improve care of the dying.[18]

6. The Institute of Medicine developed the eleven core principles for end-of-life care shown in Box 13.1. The core principles were developed by fourteen medical associations and the Joint Commission on Accreditation of Healthcare Organizations.[19]

Box 13.1. Institute of Medicine Core Principles for End-of-Life Care

- Respect the dignity of both patient and caregivers.
- Be sensitive to and respectful of the patients' and family's wishes.
- Use the most appropriate measures that are consistent with patient choices.
- Encompass alleviation of pain and other physical symptoms.
- Assess and manage psychological, social, and spiritual/religious problems.
- Offer continuity—the patient should be able to continue to be cared for, if so desired, by his or her primary care and specialist providers.
- Provide access to any therapy that may realistically be expected to improve the patient's quality of life, including alternative or nontraditional treatments.
- Provide access to palliative and hospice care.
- Respect the right to refuse treatment.
- Respect the physician's professional responsibility to discontinue some treatments when appropriate, with consideration for both patient and family preferences.
- Promote clinical- and evidence-based research on providing care at the end of life.

Source: Field, Marilyn J. and Christine K. Cassel, Eds. Approaching Death: Improving Care at the End of Life. Report of the Institute of Medicine Task Force (Washington, DC: National Academy Press, 1997).

INSTITUTE OF MEDICINE CORE PRINCIPLES
FOR END-OF-LIFE CARE

End-of-life education and support for families and patients near the end of life is an area where parish nurses may provide a valuable aspect of care. Questions for parish nurses to consider relative to the current scope of parish nursing practice are (1) Do the terms of the current *Scope and Standards of Parish Nursing Practice,* which define practice as independent practice of professional nursing, restrict parish nurses' endeavors to meet the needs of the growing number of elderly patients? (2) Should the current standards be modified to include dependent practice which would allow parish nurses to practice under MD orders, thereby enabling nurses to provide such interventions as administering immunizations and other interventions ordered by physicians to promote comfort care at end of life? Some documented needs of the elderly population include increased attention to health promotion activities. In the United States, pneumonia, influenza, and septicemia remain among the top ten killers, responsible for 5.5 percent of deaths in the sixty-five and older group. Pneumonia is now one of the most serious infections in the elderly, especially women and the oldest old.[20]

Health-promoting activities are less evident in the elderly than in the younger population. Some of the health promotion needs of the elderly population include blood pressure monitoring, cholesterol evaluations, breast and cervical cancer screening, and screening for colorectal cancer.[21] As people age, they have a higher probability of comorbidities and functional impairment. It is vital to differentiate between the physiologic effects of aging and the pathologic changes associated with chronic disease and disability. A comprehensive geriatric nursing assessment must be the basis for planning an individual health-promotion plan for a community-based older person.

PARISH NURSING PRACTICE

Parish nursing is defined as a unique, specialized practice of professional nursing that promotes health and healing within faith communities. The *Scope and Standards of Parish Nursing Practice* (1998) is based on the *Standards of Clinical Nursing Practice* (ANA, 1991), and addresses "the independent practice of professional nursing, as defined by the jurisdiction's nursing practice act, in health promotion within the context of the client's values, beliefs, and faith practices" (p. 3). The standards are in two sections: the Standards of Care and the Standards of Professional Performance. The Standards of Care section includes descriptions for standards for assessment, diagnosis, outcome identification, planning, implementation, and evaluation. The section on Standards of Professional Performance contains the descriptions of standards for quality of care, performance appraisal, education, collegiality, ethics, collaboration, research, and resource utilization.

Dependent functions of nursing practice (i.e., an intervention which may require a physician's order) are not considered within the scope of parish nursing practice. A Standard of Care (Standard IV, Planning) was developed to address the need of some clients who require care outside the independent domain of the parish nurse. Standard IV states that the health promotion plan, mutually developed with the client, "identifies the self care activities to be done by the client, the interdependence with other systems, the interventions to be performed by the parish nurse and the collaboration with, and referral to other health care professionals and providers on the basis of expected outcomes" (p. 12).

Likewise, one of the Standards for Professional Performance (Standard VI, Collaboration) states that the parish nurse collaborates with the client system, other health ministers, health care providers, and community agencies in promoting client health. A measurement criterion for the Collaboration Standard of Professional Performance is that the parish nurse consults with and refers to other health care providers as needed and integrates their expertise into the health promotion plan (p. 20).

The *Peaceful Death* competency statements were developed to assist nurse educators in incorporating end-of-life content into nursing curricula. The six competencies (1, 2, 4, 7, 11, 14) in Box 13.2, selected from the list of fifteen in the *Peaceful Death* document, are addressed from the perspective of parish nursing and in relation to current and emerging needs of persons near the end of life. Parish nurses are challenged to examine ways in which they may broaden the scope

---

Box 13.2. Selected Competencies Necessary for Nurses to Provide High-Quality Care to Patients and Families During the Transition at the End of Life

1. Recognize dynamic changes in population demographics, health care economics, and service delivery that necessitate improved professional preparation for end-of-life care.
2. Promote the provision of comfort care to the dying as an active, desirable, and important skill and an integral component of nursing care.
4. Recognize one's own attitudes, feelings, values, and expectations about death and the individual, cultural, and spiritual diversity existing in these beliefs and customs.
7. Use scientifically based standardized tools to assess symptoms, e.g., pain, dyspnea (breathlessness), constipation, anxiety, fatigue, nausea/vomiting, and altered cognition, experienced by patients at the end of life.
11. Assist the patient, family, colleagues, and oneself to cope with suffering, grief, loss, and bereavement in end-of-life care.
14. Demonstrate skill at implementing a plan for improved end-of-life care within a dynamic and complex health care delivery system.[22]

---

of practice to better provide end-of-life care and support for the growing number of elderly and their families in the community.

When an individual is nearing the end of life, one treatment option may be palliative care. The World Health Organization (WHO) defines *palliative caregivers* as those who

1. affirm life and regard dying as a normal process,
2. neither hasten nor postpone death,
3. provide relief from pain and other distressing symptoms,
4. integrate the psychological and spiritual aspects of patient care,
5. offer a support system to help patients live as actively as possible until death, and
6. offer a support system to help families cope during patients' illness and their own bereavement.[23]

Palliative care is defined as a philosophy of total care during the end-of-life period and not only includes medical treatment but also addresses the psychosocial and needs and wishes of patients and family members in an interdisciplinary manner.[24] Incorporating palliative care interventions in parish nursing plans of care may be an effective method of broadening the scope of parish nursing practice to enhance quality of life throughout the life span, and particularly at the end of life.

Quality of life issues are of great concern to elderly populations. Significant health disparity exists within the elderly population in terms of disability and access to health care as well as gender, race and ethnicity, income, education, and geographic location. Improving access to quality health services is a means for decreasing many disparities in the health and health care of the growing diverse population of older individuals. Expanding the roles of nurses providing services in the community will help to address needs of an underserved and vulnerable elderly population by improving access to care and promoting a higher quality of living and dying. Older people with health problems can remain in the community longer if nurses with appropriate skills are available in the community settings to provide or supervise care so these patients remain functional.

Jacox relates the importance of nurses having an understanding of the sociopolitical context within which they function, and the complex and interactive factors that determine who does what in health care.[25] A health care workforce does not consist of a well-defined set of roles, but changes over time in response to many factors, according to Jacox. It is influenced by the form of government within the society, definitions of health, social values, costs, the society's expectations for the health care system, and the political power of various players.

SUMMARY

This chapter presented a challenge for leaders in the field of parish nursing to reevaluate the space of parish nursing within the larger picture of the U.S. health care system. The demands for health care by Americans in the new millennium will rise disproportionately to the availability of resources. Our overburdened health care system will be forced into resource allocation issues, which have been creeping in over the past few years. Health workforce issues may require parish nurses to expand their boundaries in a specific way to include end-of-life issues in more than a counseling, education, and referral sense.

NOTES

1. Laurie A. Kamimoto, Alyssa N. Easton, Emmanuel Maurice, Corrine G. Husten, and Carol A. Macera, "Surveillance for Five Health Risks Among Older Adults—United States, 1993-1997," *MMWR,* 1999, 48(SS-8): 89-130.

2. Nadine Sahyoun, Harold Lentzner, Donna Hoyert, and Kristen N. Robinson, "Trends in Causes of Death Among the Elderly," *Centers for Disease Control and Prevention, Aging Trends,* No. 1 (Hyattsville, MD: National Center for Health Statistics, 2001), pp. 1-9.

3. Stuart J. Farber, Thomas R. Egnew, and Janet L. Herman-Bertsch, "Issues in End-of-Life Care," *The Journal of Family Practice,* 1999, 49(7): 525-530.

4. Renatta R. Loquist and Mary D. Pease, *Critical for Care: The South Carolina Nursing Workforce, 2001 and Beyond* (Columbia, SC: University of South Carolina), pp. 1-45.

5. Kenneth R. White, Patrick J. Coyne, Urvashi B. Patel, "Are Nurses Adequately Prepared for End-of-Life Care?" *Journal of Nursing Scholarship,* 2001, 33(2): 147-151.

6. Federal Agency Forum on Aging-Related Statistics (n.d.). In *Older Americans 2000: Key Indicators of Well-Being.* (Washington, DC: Government Printing Office, 2000). Health care. Retrieved June 4, 2001, from <http://www.agingstats.gov/chartbook2000/healthcare.html>.

7. Sheila Smith, Stephen K. Heffler, Stephen Calfo, Kent Clemens, Mark Freeland, Mary Lee Seifert, Arthur Sensenig, and Jean Stiller, "National Health Projections Through 2008," *Health Care Financing Review,* 1999, 21(2): 211-237.

8. Lauren A. Murray and Franklin J. Eppig, "Health Expenditures for Medicare Beneficiaries," *Health Care Financing Review,* 1999, 21(2): 281-286.

9. "Health Care Expenditures," *Older Americans 2000,* pp. 1-10.

10. Thomas A. Hodgson and Alan J. Cohen, "Medical Expenditures for Major Diseases, 1995," *Health Care Financing Review,* 1999, 21(2): 119-164.

11. Kamimoto et al., "Surveillance for Five Health Risks Among Older Adults."

12. "Health Care Expenditures," *Older Americans 2000,* pp. 1-10.

13. Health Ministries Association, Inc., and American Nurses Association, *Scope and Standards of Parish Nursing* Practice (Washington, DC: American Nurses Publishing, 1998).

14. International Council of Nurses. *Basic Principles of Nursing Care* (Washington, DC: American Nurses Publishing, 1997).

15. American Association of Colleges of Nursing, *Peaceful Death: Recommended Competencies and Curricular Guidelines for End-of-Life Nursing Care* (Washington, DC: Author, 1998). Available online <www.aacn.nche.edu/>.

16. Designing an Agenda for the Nursing Profession on End-of-Life Care: A Report of the Nursing Leadership Consortium on End-of-Life Care. Released November 1999. American Association of Critical-Care Nurses (AACN). 101 Columbia, Aliso Viejo, CA 92656; info@aacn.org; 1-800-899-2226.

17. Constance Dahlin, "Palliative Care Nursing: An Emerging Specialty," *Imprint* 47(2); 2000: 38-39.

18. <www.abcd-caring.org/action1.htm>. Accessed February 3, 2002.

19. Marilyn J. Field and Christine K. Cassel, Eds., *Approaching Death; Improving Care at the End of Life,* Report of the Institute of Medicine Task Force (Washington, DC: National Academy Press, 1997).

20. Nadine R. Sahyoun, Harold Lentzner, Donna Hoyert, and Kristen N. Robinson, "Trends in Causes of Death Among the Elderly," Centers for Disease Control, Aging Trends No. 1, National Center for Health Statistics (Hyattsville, MD: National Center for Health Statistics, 2001).

21. Gail R. Janes, Donald K. Blackman, Julie C. Bolen, Laurie A. Kamimoto, Luann Rhodes, Lee S. Caplan, Marion R. Nadel, Scott L. Tornar, James F. Lando, Stacie M. Greby, James A. Singleton, Raymond A. Strikas, and Karen G. Wooten, "Surveillance for Use of Preventive Health-Care Services by Older Adults, 1995-1997," *MMWR,* 1999, 48(SS-8): 51-88.

22. American Association of Colleges of Nursing, *Peaceful Death.*

23. White, Coyne, and Patel, "Are Nurses Adequately Prepared for End-of-Life Care?"

24. Ruth McCorkle and Jeannie V. Pasacreta, "Enhancing Caregiver Outcomes in Palliative Care." *Cancer Control: JMCC,* 2001, 8(1): 36-45.

25. Ada Jacox, "Determinants of Who Does What in Health Care," *Online Journal of Issues in Nursing* (December 30, 1997). Available <http://www.nursingworld.org/ojin/tpc5/tpc5_1.htm>.

Index

Page numbers followed by the letter "b" indicate boxed material; those followed by the letter "f" indicate figures; and those followed by the letter "t" indicate tables.

SPECIAL 25%-OFF DISCOUNT!
Order a copy of this book with this form or online at:
http://www.haworthpressinc.com/store/product.asp?sku=4815

PARISH NURSING
A Handbook for the New Millennium

_____in hardbound at $44.96 (regularly $59.95) (ISBN: 0-7890-1817-9)

_____in softbound at $22.46 (regularly $29.95) (ISBN: 0-7890-1818-7)

Or order online and use Code HEC25 in the shopping cart.

COST OF BOOKS_____	☐ **BILL ME LATER:** ($5 service charge will be added)
OUTSIDE US/CANADA/ MEXICO: ADD 20%_____	(Bill-me option is good on US/Canada/Mexico orders only; not good to jobbers, wholesalers, or subscription agencies.)
POSTAGE & HANDLING_____ *(US: $5.00 for first book & $2.00 for each additional book) Outside US: $6.00 for first book & $2.00 for each additional book)*	☐ Check here if billing address is different from shipping address and attach purchase order and billing address information. Signature_____
SUBTOTAL_____	☐ **PAYMENT ENCLOSED: $**_____
IN CANADA: ADD 7% GST_____	☐ **PLEASE CHARGE TO MY CREDIT CARD.**
STATE TAX_____ *(NY, OH & MN residents, please add appropriate local sales tax)*	☐ Visa ☐ MasterCard ☐ AmEx ☐ Discover ☐ Diner's Club ☐ Eurocard ☐ JCB Account # _____
FINAL TOTAL_____ *(If paying in Canadian funds, convert using the current exchange rate, UNESCO coupons welcome)*	Exp. Date_____ Signature_____

Prices in US dollars and subject to change without notice.

NAME_____

INSTITUTION_____

ADDRESS_____

CITY_____

STATE/ZIP_____

COUNTRY_____ COUNTY (NY residents only)_____

TEL_____ FAX_____

E-MAIL_____

May we use your e-mail address for confirmations and other types of information? ☐ Yes ☐ No
We appreciate receiving your e-mail address and fax number. Haworth would like to e-mail or fax special discount offers to you, as a preferred customer. **We will never share, rent, or exchange your e-mail address or fax number.** We regard such actions as an invasion of your privacy.

Order From Your Local Bookstore or Directly From
The Haworth Press, Inc.
10 Alice Street, Binghamton, New York 13904-1580 • USA
TELEPHONE: 1-800-HAWORTH (1-800-429-6784) / Outside US/Canada: (607) 722-5857
FAX: 1-800-895-0582 / Outside US/Canada: (607) 722-6362
E-mail to: getinfo@haworthpressinc.com
PLEASE PHOTOCOPY THIS FORM FOR YOUR PERSONAL USE.
http://www.HaworthPress.com   BOF02